-The C

KETO DIET COOKBOOK

FOR BEGINNERS 2024

1200 Days of Delicious Recipes made with Low- Carb to Lose Weight with 30-Day Meal Plan

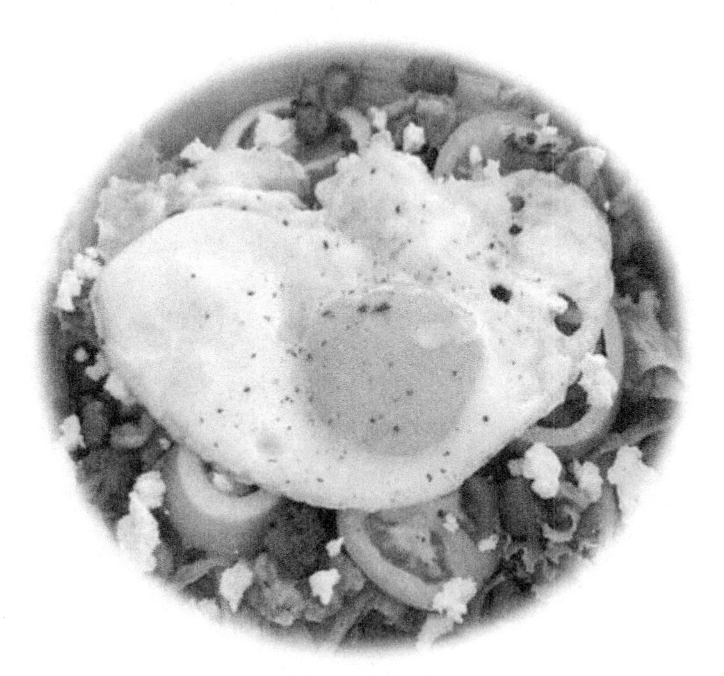

DR. SANDRA T. CADWELL

This cookbook is a work of non-fiction. The recipes, tips, and advice provided are based on the author's experiences and research.

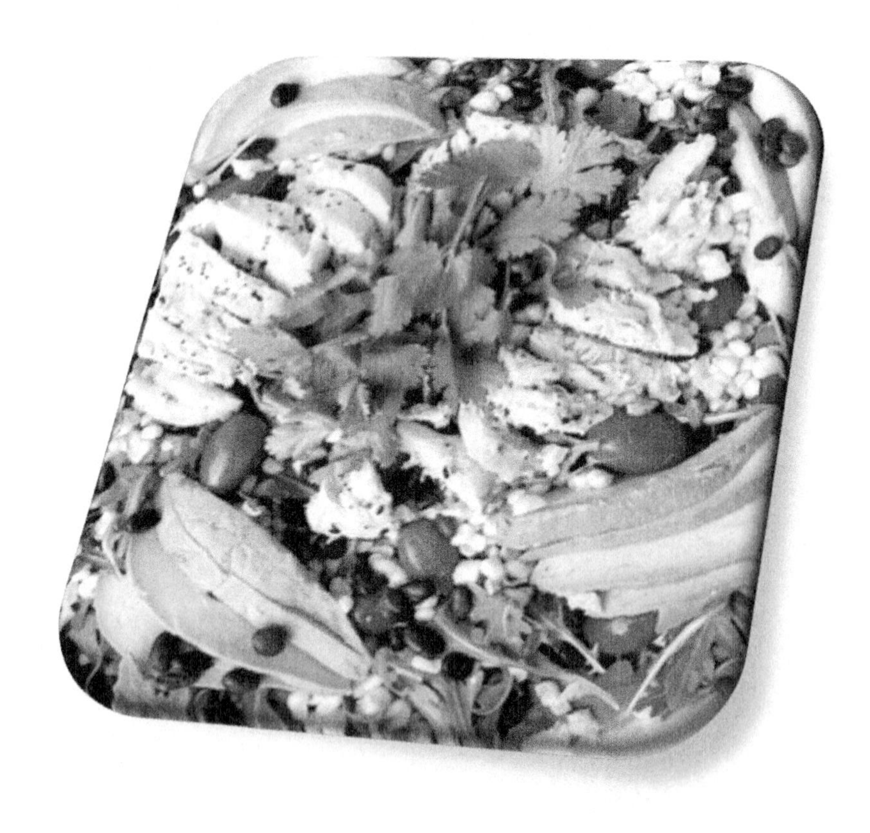

TABLE OF CONTENTS

INTRODUCTION

Sarah, at the age of fifty-seven, felt at a crossroads. The years had passed, leaving traces of laughter, love, and life events carved in the creases of her face. But along with those memories came the unavoidable truth: her health wasn't what it used to be. Her energy levels were dwindling, her weight appeared to be steadily increasing, and her doctor had gently reminded her of the need of taking care of herself as she approached her golden years.

Sarah had always been optimistic, believing in the potential of change and progress. So when she came across "The Complete Keto Diet Cookbook for Beginners 2024" on one of her late-night online searches, something inside her sparked. It was as if the cosmos had whispered to her, offering her the opportunity for transformation and rejuvenation.

She dived into the cookbook with curiosity and conviction. As she read about the ketogenic diet, with its emphasis on low-carb, high-fat meals and possible advantages for weight reduction and overall health, she felt a spark of hope flare inside her. Maybe, just maybe, this may be the secret to regaining her vibrancy and enthusiasm for life.

Sarah began her keto adventure, guided by the cookbook. She cleaned out her cabinet of sugary snacks and processed meals, replacing them with fresh veggies, lean meats, and healthy fats. With excellent recipes and a new sense of purpose, she returned to the kitchen with a revitalized zest for cooking.

The days grew into weeks, and Sarah found herself enjoying the pleasure of preparing meals that not only nourished her body but also thrilled her taste senses. She found the beauty of cauliflower rice, the adaptability of zucchini noodles, and the rich flavor of avocado-based dishes. Each dish she attempted seemed like a minor win, bringing her closer to her goal of improved health and vigor.

Sarah noted tiny changes in her physique over the course of many weeks. The excess weight she had carried for years began to peel away, exposing a smaller, more toned form beneath. Her energy levels skyrocketed, allowing her to face her days with fresh zeal and zest. Perhaps most significantly, she felt a sense of strength that she hadn't had in years, knowing that she was taking charge of her health one meal at a time.

However, Sarah's keto journey had benefits that extended beyond the physical. She felt more confident, radiant, and vibrant than she had in decades. Gone were the days of self-doubt and uneasiness; in their stead stood a lady who understood her value and accepted her age with elegance and dignity.

And as Sarah proceeded on her keto quest, she couldn't help but be pleased for coming upon "The Complete Keto Diet Cookbook for Beginners 2024". It was more than simply a compilation of recipes; it was a guide to a better, happier existence. It served as a reminder that, regardless of your age or circumstances, it is never too late to make a change and rewrite the tale of your health and vitality.

So, if you ever find yourself at a crossroads, as Sarah did months ago, remember that you have the ability to improve your life. And with the correct tools, mentality, and support, everything is achievable. So, why wait? Begin your keto adventure now and uncover the great potential within you.

CHAPTER ONE

Understanding the Keto Diet

Few dietary trends and weight reduction regimens have sparked as much interest and curiosity as the ketogenic diet, or keto for short. To appreciate its significance, we must take a tour into our bodies' complicated workings, investigating the metabolic phenomena known as ketosis and its tremendous influence on weight reduction and health.

The ketogenic diet is a high-fat, moderate-protein, low-carbohydrate eating plan that aims to change the body's metabolism away from depending on glucose for fuel and toward burning fat for energy. This metabolic condition, known as ketosis, is accomplished by significantly lowering carbohydrate intake while increasing consumption of healthy fats and maintaining a moderate protein intake.

The Mechanism of Ketosis

To understand the magic of the keto diet, we must first unravel the complicated metabolic processes that occur within the body. Under normal circumstances, carbohydrates are broken down into glucose, the body's major source of energy. However, in the absence of carbs, such as during fasting or extreme carbohydrate restriction, the body experiences a metabolic change.

In ketosis, the liver starts producing molecules called ketones from stored fat, which act as an alternate fuel source for the brain and body. Ketones can pass the blood-brain barrier, giving a constant source of energy to the brain while eliminating the need for glucose.

This change from glucose to ketones as the predominant fuel source is a characteristic of ketosis and is crucial to the ketogenic diet's effectiveness.

The Impact on Weight Loss

One of the most appealing characteristics of the ketogenic diet is its propensity to stimulate weight reduction, frequently with dramatic results. By limiting carbohydrate consumption and causing ketosis, the body becomes extremely effective at burning fat for fuel, both from food sources and stored body fat. This results in a reduction in both body weight and body fat percentage, particularly visceral fat, which has been linked to a variety of health hazards, including cardiovascular disease and type 2 diabetes.

Furthermore, ketosis has been found to lower hunger and improve feelings of fullness, resulting in natural calorie reduction without the need for stringent portion control or calorie tracking. Furthermore, the ketogenic diet has been associated to positive hormonal changes, including higher levels of the satiety hormone leptin and lower levels of the hunger hormone ghrelin, which aids in weight reduction attempts.

Understanding Macronutrients on Keto

The ketogenic diet's effectiveness is dependent on careful adjustment of macronutrients, which are the three major components of our diet: fat, protein, and carbs. Individuals can improve their metabolic status and get the benefits of ketosis by deliberately altering the macronutrient ratios.

Fat: The Primary Energy Source

Contrary to traditional nutritional thinking, fat takes center stage on the ketogenic diet, accounting for the bulk of calorie intake. Avocados, nuts, seeds, olive oil, and fatty fish are high in energy and help to maintain ketosis. Fats not only give long-lasting energy, but they also enhance satiety and the absorption of fat-soluble vitamins.

Protein: Building Blocks of Muscle

While fat reigns supreme on the ketogenic diet, protein is also an essential component, acting as the foundation for muscle repair and development. However, it is critical to establish a balance since excessive protein ingestion has the potential to impair ketosis by boosting glucose synthesis through a process called gluconeogenesis. Choose moderate portions of high-quality protein sources including poultry, fish, eggs, and tofu to promote muscular health while staying keto.

Carbohydrates: The Key to Ketosis

In striking contrast to standard dietary guidelines, carbohydrates are strictly limited on the ketogenic diet, accounting for less than 5-10% of total calorie intake. Individuals who limit their carbohydrate intake can efficiently deplete glycogen reserves and enter ketosis, in which fat becomes the predominant fuel source. Concentrate on fiber, nutrient-dense carbohydrate sources such as leafy greens, cruciferous vegetables, and berries, which supply critical vitamins, minerals, and antioxidants while maintaining ketosis.

Calculating and Tracking Macros

Achieving and sustaining ketosis necessitates exact macronutrient calculation and tracking. Numerous online calculators and mobile applications are available to help people discover their appropriate macronutrient ratios depending on age, gender, weight, exercise level, and intended goals.

Determining Your Macros

To calculate your specific macronutrient objectives, first determine your daily calorie requirements based on your basal metabolic rate (BMR) and activity level. From there, assign a proportion of calories to each macronutrient category, which normally ranges between 70-80% fat, 20-25% protein, and 5-10% carbs. Adjust these ratios as required based on personal preferences, metabolic reaction, and objectives.

Tracking Your Progress

When it comes to the ketogenic diet, consistency is essential, and meticulous macronutrient monitoring may give crucial insights into your progress and adherence to the plan.

To document your meals, use food tracking apps or notebooks and record the grams of fat, protein, and carbs ingested throughout the day. Regularly review your progress, making modifications as needed to ensure that you stay within your target macronutrient levels and continue to benefit from ketosis.

The ketogenic diet offers a paradigm change in our understanding of nutrition and metabolic health, providing an effective tool for weight loss, increased energy, and general well-being.Individuals who embrace ketosis principles and understand macronutrient manipulation can unlock the ketogenic diet's transforming potential and begin on a journey to optimal health and vigor.

CHAPTER TWO

Breakfast Recipes

Keto Avocado and Bacon Egg Cups

Prep Time: 10 minutes

Cooking Time: 20 minutes

Servings: 4

Ingredients:

- 4 large eggs
- 2 ripe avocados
- 4 slices of bacon
- Salt and pepper to taste
- Fresh chives or parsley for garnish (optional)

Method of Preparation:

1. Preheat your oven to 375°F (190°C) and lightly grease a muffin tin with cooking spray.
2. Cut the avocados in half and remove the pits. Scoop out a small portion of avocado flesh from each half to create a larger well for the egg.
3. Place the avocado halves in the muffin tin, ensuring they are stable and level.
4. Crack one egg into each avocado half, being careful not to overflow.
5. Season each egg with salt and pepper to taste.
6. Cut the bacon slices in half and wrap each avocado half with a bacon slice, securing it around the avocado.
7. Bake in the preheated oven for 15-20 minutes or until the egg whites are set and the bacon is crispy.

8. Remove from the oven and garnish with fresh chives or parsley if desired.
9. Serve hot and enjoy!

Nutritional Info (per serving):
Calories: 257 | Total Fat: 21g | Saturated Fat: 5g | Cholesterol: 193mg | Sodium: 228mg | Total Carbohydrates: 5g | Dietary Fiber: 3g | Sugars: 0g | Protein: 11g

Recipe Name: ______________________

Date: / / ***Time:*** _____

Rating: ☆☆☆☆☆

S/N	Ingredients	Adjustment

Cooking Experience: ______________________

____

____

____

Notes: ______________________

____

____

____

____

____

____

____

Keto Chia Seed Pudding

Prep Time: 5 minutes (plus overnight chilling)

Cooking Time: 0 minutes

Servings: 2

Ingredients:

- 1/4 cup chia seeds
- 1 cup unsweetened almond milk
- 1 tablespoon unsweetened cocoa powder
- 1/2 teaspoon vanilla extract
- 1-2 tablespoons keto-friendly sweetener (such as erythritol or stevia), to taste
- **Optional toppings:** fresh berries, unsweetened coconut flakes, chopped nuts

Method of Preparation:

1. In a mixing bowl, combine the chia seeds, almond milk, cocoa powder, vanilla extract, and keto-friendly sweetener. Mix well to ensure the cocoa powder is fully incorporated.
2. Let the mixture sit for 5 minutes, then whisk again to prevent clumping.
3. Cover the bowl and refrigerate overnight or for at least 4 hours to allow the chia seeds to absorb the liquid and thicken into a pudding-like consistency.
4. Once chilled and thickened, give the pudding a final stir to ensure an even texture.
5. Divide the chia seed pudding into serving bowls or glasses.
6. Garnish with your choice of toppings, such as fresh berries, unsweetened coconut flakes, or chopped nuts.
7. Serve chilled and enjoy!

Nutritional Info (per serving):
Calories: 144 | Total Fat: 9g | Saturated Fat: 1g | Cholesterol: 0mg | Sodium: 89mg | Total Carbohydrates: 15g | Dietary Fiber: 10g | Sugars: 1g | Protein: 5g

Recipe Name:____________________

Date: / /   ***Time:***____

Rating: ☆☆☆☆☆

S/N	Ingredients	Adjustment

Cooking Experience: ____________________

____

____

____

Notes:____________________

____

____

____

____

____

____

____

Keto Spinach and Feta Omelette

Prep Time: 5 minutes

Cooking Time: 10 minutes

Servings: 1

Ingredients:

- 3 large eggs
- 1/4 cup fresh spinach, chopped
- 2 tablespoons crumbled feta cheese
- 1 tablespoon unsalted butter or olive oil
- Salt and pepper to taste

Method of Preparation:

1. In a small bowl, beat the eggs until well combined. Season with salt and pepper to taste.
2. Heat the butter or olive oil in a non-stick skillet over medium heat.
3. Add the chopped spinach to the skillet and sauté for 1-2 minutes until wilted.
4. Pour the beaten eggs over the spinach, swirling the skillet to ensure an even distribution.
5. Cook the omelette for 2-3 minutes, gently lifting the edges with a spatula to allow the uncooked eggs to flow underneath.
6. Once the eggs are mostly set, sprinkle the crumbled feta cheese evenly over one half of the omelette.
7. Carefully fold the other half of the omelette over the filling to create a half-moon shape.
8. Cook for another 1-2 minutes until the cheese is melted and the omelette is cooked through.

9. Slide the omelette onto a plate, cut in half if desired, and serve hot.
10. Enjoy your delicious keto spinach and feta omelette!

Nutritional Info (per serving):
Calories: 321 | Total Fat: 26g | Saturated Fat: 12g | Cholesterol: 568mg | Sodium: 405mg | Total Carbohydrates: 2g | Dietary Fiber: 1g | Sugars: 0g | Protein: 19g

Recipe Name:______________________

Date: / / ***Time:*____**

Rating: ☆☆☆☆☆

S/N	Ingredients	Adjustment

Cooking Experience: ______________________________

____

____

____

Notes:______________________________

____

____

____

____

____

____

____

Keto Coconut Flour Pancakes

Prep Time: 10 minutes

Cooking Time: 10 minutes

Servings: 2

Ingredients:

- 2 large eggs
- 1/4 cup unsweetened almond milk
- 2 tablespoons coconut flour
- 1 tablespoon keto-friendly sweetener (such as erythritol or stevia)
- 1/2 teaspoon baking powder
- 1/4 teaspoon vanilla extract
- Pinch of salt
- Butter or coconut oil for cooking
- **Optional toppings:** sugar-free maple syrup, berries, whipped cream

Method of Preparation:

1. In a mixing bowl, whisk together the eggs, almond milk, vanilla extract, and keto-friendly sweetener until well combined.
2. In a separate bowl, sift together the coconut flour, baking powder, and salt.
3. Gradually add the dry ingredients to the wet ingredients, whisking until a smooth batter forms. Let the batter rest for 5 minutes to allow the coconut flour to absorb the liquid.
4. Heat a non-stick skillet or griddle over medium heat and lightly grease with butter or coconut oil.
5. Pour 1/4 cup of batter onto the skillet to form each pancake, spreading it out slightly with the back of a spoon.

6. Cook the pancakes for 2-3 minutes on one side until bubbles form on the surface, then flip and cook for an additional 1-2 minutes on the other side until golden brown and cooked through.
7. Repeat with the remaining batter, adjusting the heat as needed to prevent burning.
8. Serve the coconut flour pancakes hot with your choice of toppings, such as sugar-free maple syrup, berries, or whipped cream.
9. Enjoy your fluffy and delicious keto-friendly pancakes!

Nutritional Info (per serving, without toppings):
Calories: 144 | Total Fat: 9g | Saturated Fat: 4g | Cholesterol: 186mg | Sodium: 233mg | Total Carbohydrates: 7g | Dietary Fiber: 4g | Sugars: 1g | Protein: 7g

Recipe Name:______________________________

Date: / / ***Time:***_____

Rating: ☆☆☆☆☆

S/N	Ingredients	Adjustment

Cooking Experience: ______________________________

____

____

____

Notes:______________________________

____

____

____

____

____

____

____

Keto Breakfast Casserole

Prep Time: 10 minutes
Cooking Time: 30 minutes
Servings: 6
Ingredients:

- 8 large eggs
- 1/2 cup unsweetened almond milk
- 1 cup shredded cheddar cheese
- 1 cup chopped broccoli florets
- 1/2 cup diced bell peppers (any color)
- 4 slices cooked bacon, crumbled
- 2 tablespoons chopped fresh chives
- Salt and pepper to taste
- Cooking spray or butter for greasing

Method of Preparation:

1. Preheat your oven to 375°F (190°C). Grease a 9x9-inch baking dish with cooking spray or butter.
2. In a large mixing bowl, whisk together the eggs and almond milk until well combined. Season with salt and pepper to taste.
3. Stir in the shredded cheddar cheese, chopped broccoli florets, diced bell peppers, crumbled bacon, and chopped fresh chives until evenly distributed.
4. Pour the egg mixture into the prepared baking dish, spreading it out evenly.
5. Bake in the preheated oven for 25-30 minutes or until the eggs are set and the top is golden brown.
6. Remove from the oven and let cool for a few minutes before slicing into squares or rectangles.

7. Serve hot and enjoy your hearty keto breakfast casserole!

Nutritional Info (per serving):
Calories: 231 | Total Fat: 17g | Saturated Fat: 7g | Cholesterol: 286mg | Sodium: 371mg | Total Carbohydrates: 4g | Dietary Fiber: 1g | Sugars: 1g | Protein: 16g

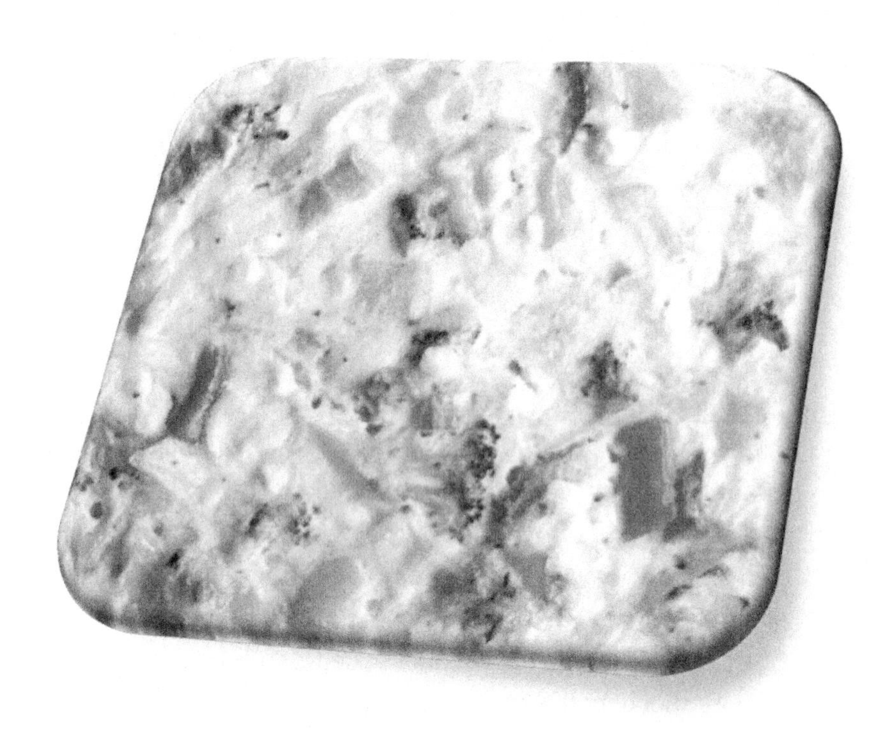

Recipe Name:______________________________

Date: / / ***Time:***_____

Rating: ☆☆☆☆☆

S/N	Ingredients	Adjustment

Cooking Experience: ______________________________

____

____

____

Notes:______________________________________

____

____

____

____

____

____

____

Keto Green Smoothie Bowl

Prep Time: 5 minutes

Cooking Time: 0 minutes

Servings: 1

Ingredients:

- 1 cup unsweetened almond milk or coconut milk
- 1/2 avocado, peeled and pitted
- 1 cup fresh spinach leaves
- 1/2 cup chopped cucumber
- 1/4 cup chopped celery
- 1/4 cup fresh parsley or cilantro leaves
- Juice of 1/2 lime
- 1 tablespoon chia seeds
- **Optional toppings:** sliced strawberries, unsweetened coconut flakes, chopped nuts

Method of Preparation:

1. In a blender, combine the unsweetened almond milk, avocado, spinach leaves, chopped cucumber, chopped celery, fresh parsley or cilantro leaves, lime juice, and chia seeds.
2. Blend on high speed until smooth and creamy, adding more almond milk if needed to reach your desired consistency.
3. Pour the green smoothie into a bowl.
4. Top with sliced strawberries, unsweetened coconut flakes, and chopped nuts if desired.
5. Serve immediately and enjoy your refreshing keto green smoothie bowl!

Nutritional Info (per serving, without toppings):
Calories: 224 | Total Fat: 16g | Saturated Fat: 2g | Cholesterol: 0mg | Sodium: 181mg | Total Carbohydrates: 14g | Dietary Fiber: 9g | Sugars: 1g | Protein: 6g

Recipe Name:______________________________

Date: / /   ***Time:***_____

Rating: ☆☆☆☆☆

S/N	Ingredients	Adjustment

Cooking Experience: ______________________________

____

____

____

Notes:______________________________

____

____

____

____

____

____

____

Keto Mushroom and Cheese Frittata

Prep Time: 10 minutes

Cooking Time: 20 minutes

Servings: 4

Ingredients:

- 8 large eggs
- 1/4 cup heavy cream or full-fat coconut milk
- 1 cup sliced mushrooms
- 1/2 cup shredded Swiss cheese
- 2 tablespoons chopped fresh parsley
- 1 tablespoon unsalted butter or olive oil
- Salt and pepper to taste

Method of Preparation:

1. Preheat your oven to 350°F (175°C).
2. In a mixing bowl, whisk together the eggs and heavy cream or coconut milk until well combined. Season with salt and pepper to taste.
3. Heat the butter or olive oil in an oven-safe skillet over medium heat.
4. Add the sliced mushrooms to the skillet and sauté for 3-4 minutes until they begin to soften.
5. Pour the egg mixture into the skillet, swirling to evenly distribute the mushrooms.
6. Sprinkle the shredded Swiss cheese over the top of the egg mixture.
7. Transfer the skillet to the preheated oven and bake for 15-20 minutes until the frittata is set in the center and the edges are golden brown.

8. Remove from the oven and sprinkle with chopped fresh parsley.
9. Slice the frittata into wedges and serve hot.
10. Enjoy your flavorful keto mushroom and cheese frittata!

Nutritional Info (per serving):
Calories: 239 | Total Fat: 18g | Saturated Fat: 9g | Cholesterol: 363mg | Sodium: 255mg | Total Carbohydrates: 3g | Dietary Fiber: 1g | Sugars: 1g | Protein: 16g

Recipe Name:____________________

Date: / /

Time:____

Rating: ☆☆☆☆☆

S/N	Ingredients	Adjustment

Cooking Experience: ____________________

____

____

____

Notes:____________________

____

____

____

____

____

____

____

Keto Almond Flour Waffles

Prep Time: 10 minutes

Cooking Time: 10 minutes

Servings: 2

Ingredients:

- 1 cup almond flour
- 2 large eggs
- 1/4 cup unsweetened almond milk
- 2 tablespoons melted coconut oil or unsalted butter
- 1 tablespoon keto-friendly sweetener (such as erythritol or stevia)
- 1 teaspoon baking powder
- 1/2 teaspoon vanilla extract
- Pinch of salt
- Cooking spray or additional coconut oil for greasing

Method of Preparation:

1. Preheat your waffle iron according to the manufacturer's instructions.
2. In a mixing bowl, whisk together the almond flour, baking powder, keto-friendly sweetener, and salt until well combined.
3. In a separate bowl, beat the eggs until frothy. Stir in the unsweetened almond milk, melted coconut oil or butter, and vanilla extract.
4. Gradually add the wet ingredients to the dry ingredients, stirring until a smooth batter forms.
5. Lightly grease the waffle iron with cooking spray or coconut oil.

6. Pour the batter onto the preheated waffle iron, spreading it out evenly.
7. Close the waffle iron and cook for 4-5 minutes until the waffles are golden brown and crisp.
8. Carefully remove the waffles from the iron and repeat with the remaining batter.
9. Serve the almond flour waffles hot with your favorite keto-friendly toppings, such as sugar-free maple syrup, whipped cream, or berries.
10. Enjoy your fluffy and delicious keto waffles!

Nutritional Info (per serving, without toppings):
Calories: 361 | Total Fat: 32g | Saturated Fat: 13g | Cholesterol: 186mg | Sodium: 199mg | Total Carbohydrates: 8g | Dietary Fiber: 4g | Sugars: 1g | Protein: 13g

Recipe Name: ______________________________

Date: / /

Time: _____

Rating: ☆☆☆☆☆

S/N	Ingredients	Adjustment

Cooking Experience: ______________________________

____

____

____

Notes: ______________________________

____

____

____

____

____

____

____

Keto Sausage and Egg Muffins

Prep Time: 10 minutes
Cooking Time: 20 minutes
Servings: 6
Ingredients:

- 6 large eggs
- 1/4 cup heavy cream or full-fat coconut milk
- 1/2 cup shredded cheddar cheese
- 6 cooked breakfast sausage patties, chopped
- 1/4 cup chopped bell peppers (any color)
- 1/4 cup chopped onions
- Salt and pepper to taste
- Cooking spray or butter for greasing

Method of Preparation:

1. Preheat your oven to 375°F (190°C). Grease a 6-cup muffin tin with cooking spray or butter.
2. In a mixing bowl, whisk together the eggs and heavy cream or coconut milk until well combined. Season with salt and pepper to taste.
3. Stir in the shredded cheddar cheese, chopped breakfast sausage patties, chopped bell peppers, and chopped onions until evenly distributed.
4. Pour the egg mixture into the prepared muffin tin, filling each cup about 2/3 full.
5. Bake in the preheated oven for 15-20 minutes until the egg muffins are set and lightly golden brown on top.
6. Remove from the oven and let cool for a few minutes before removing the egg muffins from the tin.

7. Serve hot or let cool completely before storing in an airtight container in the refrigerator.
8. Enjoy your portable and protein-packed keto sausage and egg muffins for a satisfying breakfast on the go!

Nutritional Info (per serving):
Calories: 242 | Total Fat: 20g | Saturated Fat: 9g | Cholesterol: 248mg | Sodium: 411mg | Total Carbohydrates: 2g | Dietary Fiber: 0g | Sugars: 1g | Protein: 13g

Recipe Name:______________________

Date: / / ***Time:***_____

Rating: ☆☆☆☆☆

S/N	Ingredients	Adjustment

Cooking Experience: ______________________________

____

____

____

Notes:______________________________

____

____

____

____

____

____

____

Keto Greek Yogurt Parfait

Prep Time: 5 minutes
Cooking Time: 0 minutes
Servings: 1
Ingredients:

- 1/2 cup full-fat Greek yogurt
- 1/4 cup fresh berries (such as strawberries, blueberries, or raspberries)
- 1 tablespoon unsweetened coconut flakes
- 1 tablespoon chopped nuts (such as almonds, walnuts, or pecans)
- 1 tablespoon chia seeds or ground flaxseeds
- 1 tablespoon keto-friendly sweetener (such as erythritol or stevia), optional
- Dash of cinnamon or vanilla extract, optional

Method of Preparation:

1. In a serving glass or bowl, layer the full-fat Greek yogurt, fresh berries, unsweetened coconut flakes, chopped nuts, and chia seeds or ground flaxseeds.
2. If desired, sprinkle with keto-friendly sweetener and a dash of cinnamon or vanilla extract for extra flavor.
3. Repeat the layering process until all ingredients are used, ending with a final layer of yogurt on top.
4. Serve immediately and enjoy your creamy and satisfying keto Greek yogurt parfait!

Nutritional Info (per serving):
Calories: 247 | Total Fat: 15g | Saturated Fat: 9g | Cholesterol: 10mg | Sodium: 28mg | Total Carbohydrates: 14g | Dietary Fiber: 6g | Sugars: 6g | Protein: 17g

Recipe Name:____________________________

Date: / / ***Time:*_____**

Rating: ☆☆☆☆☆

S/N	Ingredients	Adjustment

Cooking Experience: ____________________________________

Notes:____

CHAPTER THREE

Lunch Recipes

Keto Chicken and Avocado Salad

Prep Time: 10 minutes
Cooking Time: 10 minutes
Servings: 2
Ingredients:

- 2 boneless, skinless chicken breasts
- 1 tablespoon olive oil
- Salt and pepper to taste
- 4 cups mixed salad greens (such as spinach, arugula, and romaine)
- 1 avocado, diced
- 1/4 cup cherry tomatoes, halved
- 1/4 cup cucumber, sliced
- 2 tablespoons crumbled feta cheese
- 2 tablespoons sliced almonds
- Keto-friendly salad dressing of choice (such as balsamic vinaigrette or ranch)

Method of Preparation:

1. Season the chicken breasts with salt and pepper on both sides.
2. In a skillet over medium-high heat, heat the olive oil. Add the chicken breasts and cook for 4-5 minutes per side until cooked through and golden brown. Remove from the skillet and let rest for a few minutes before slicing.

3. In a large bowl, combine the mixed salad greens, diced avocado, halved cherry tomatoes, sliced cucumber, crumbled feta cheese, and sliced almonds.
4. Add the sliced chicken breasts to the salad.
5. Drizzle the salad with your choice of keto-friendly salad dressing and toss gently to coat.
6. Divide the salad between two plates and serve immediately.
7. Enjoy your refreshing and satisfying keto chicken and avocado salad!

Nutritional Info (per serving):
Calories: 418 | Total Fat: 27g | Saturated Fat: 5g | Cholesterol: 81mg | Sodium: 244mg | Total Carbohydrates: 13g | Dietary Fiber: 8g | Sugars: 2g | Protein: 32g

Recipe Name:______________________

Date: / / ***Time:***_____

Rating: ☆☆☆☆☆

S/N	Ingredients	Adjustment

Cooking Experience: ______________________________

Notes:______________________________

Keto Zucchini Noodles with Pesto and Cherry Tomatoes

Prep Time: 15 minutes

Cooking Time: 10 minutes

Servings: 2

Ingredients:

- 2 medium zucchinis, spiralized into noodles
- 1 tablespoon olive oil
- 2 tablespoons keto-friendly pesto sauce
- 1 cup cherry tomatoes, halved
- 2 tablespoons grated Parmesan cheese
- Salt and pepper to taste
- Fresh basil leaves for garnish (optional)

Method of Preparation:

1. Heat the olive oil in a skillet over medium heat.
2. Add the spiralized zucchini noodles to the skillet and sauté for 3-4 minutes until tender.
3. Stir in the keto-friendly pesto sauce and halved cherry tomatoes, tossing gently to coat.
4. Cook for an additional 2-3 minutes until the cherry tomatoes are slightly softened.
5. Season the zucchini noodles with salt and pepper to taste.
6. Divide the zucchini noodles between two plates.
7. Sprinkle with grated Parmesan cheese and garnish with fresh basil leaves if desired.
8. Serve hot and enjoy your flavorful and nutritious keto zucchini noodles with pesto and cherry tomatoes!

Nutritional Info (per serving):
Calories: 215 | Total Fat: 16g | Saturated Fat: 3g | Cholesterol: 4mg | Sodium: 227mg | Total Carbohydrates: 10g | Dietary Fiber: 3g | Sugars: 5g | Protein: 6g

Recipe Name:______________________

Date: / /   ***Time:***_____

Rating: ☆☆☆☆☆

S/N	Ingredients	Adjustment

Cooking Experience: ______________________

____

____

____

Notes:______________________

____

____

____

____

____

____

____

Keto Turkey and Cheese Lettuce Wraps

Prep Time: 10 minutes
Cooking Time: 0 minutes
Servings: 2
Ingredients:

- 8 large lettuce leaves (such as iceberg or butter lettuce)
- 8 slices turkey breast
- 4 slices Swiss cheese
- 1/2 avocado, sliced
- 1/4 cup sliced red bell pepper
- 1/4 cup sliced cucumber
- 1/4 cup shredded carrots
- Keto-friendly mustard or mayonnaise, optional
- Salt and pepper to taste

Method of Preparation:

1. Lay out the lettuce leaves on a clean work surface.
2. Layer two slices of turkey breast, one slice of Swiss cheese, avocado slices, red bell pepper slices, cucumber slices, and shredded carrots on each lettuce leaf.
3. If desired, spread a thin layer of keto-friendly mustard or mayonnaise on top of the fillings.
4. Season with salt and pepper to taste.
5. Roll up the lettuce leaves tightly to form wraps.
6. Secure the wraps with toothpicks if needed.
7. Serve immediately and enjoy your delicious and satisfying keto turkey and cheese lettuce wraps!

Nutritional Info (per serving):
Calories: 273 | Total Fat: 18g | Saturated Fat: 6g | Cholesterol: 49mg | Sodium: 468mg | Total Carbohydrates: 9g | Dietary Fiber: 4g | Sugars: 3g | Protein: 21g

Recipe Name:________________________

Date: / /   ***Time:***____

Rating: ☆☆☆☆☆

S/N	Ingredients	Adjustment

Cooking Experience: ______________________________

Notes:____________________________________

Keto Cauliflower Fried Rice

Prep Time: 15 minutes

Cooking Time: 15 minutes

Servings: 4

Ingredients:

- 1 medium head cauliflower, riced (or 4 cups pre-riced cauliflower)
- 2 tablespoons coconut oil or olive oil
- 2 cloves garlic, minced
- 1 tablespoon grated ginger
- 1/2 cup diced onion
- 1/2 cup diced bell peppers (any color)
- 1/2 cup diced carrots
- 1/2 cup diced broccoli florets
- 2 large eggs, beaten
- 2 tablespoons soy sauce or tamari (for gluten-free)
- 1 tablespoon sesame oil
- 2 green onions, thinly sliced
- Salt and pepper to taste

Method of Preparation:

1. In a large skillet or wok, heat the coconut oil or olive oil over medium heat.
2. Add the minced garlic and grated ginger to the skillet and sauté for 1 minute until fragrant.
3. Add the diced onion, bell peppers, carrots, and broccoli florets to the skillet. Cook for 5-7 minutes until the vegetables are tender-crisp.

4. Push the vegetables to one side of the skillet and pour the beaten eggs into the empty space. Scramble the eggs until cooked through, then stir to combine with the vegetables.
5. Add the riced cauliflower to the skillet, stirring to combine with the vegetables and eggs.
6. Drizzle the soy sauce or tamari and sesame oil over the cauliflower fried rice. Stir well to evenly distribute the sauces.
7. Cook for an additional 3-5 minutes, stirring occasionally, until the cauliflower is tender and heated through.
8. Season with salt and pepper to taste.
9. Garnish with thinly sliced green onions before serving.
10. Enjoy your flavorful and nutritious keto cauliflower fried rice as a satisfying lunch option!

Nutritional Info (per serving):
Calories: 152 | Total Fat: 10g | Saturated Fat: 5g | Cholesterol: 93mg | Sodium: 489mg | Total Carbohydrates: 11g | Dietary Fiber: 4g | Sugars: 5g | Protein: 7g

Recipe Name:___________________________

Date: / /

Time:_____

Rating: ☆☆☆☆☆

S/N	Ingredients	Adjustment

Cooking Experience: ___________________________

____

____

____

Notes:___________________________

____

____

____

____

____

____

____

Keto Chicken Caesar Salad

Prep Time: 15 minutes

Cooking Time: 15 minutes

Servings: 2

Ingredients:

- 2 boneless, skinless chicken breasts
- 1 tablespoon olive oil
- Salt and pepper to taste
- 6 cups chopped romaine lettuce
- 1/4 cup grated Parmesan cheese
- 1/4 cup Caesar dressing (keto-friendly)
- 1/4 cup keto-friendly croutons (optional)

Method of Preparation:

1. Season the chicken breasts with salt and pepper on both sides.
2. Heat the olive oil in a skillet over medium-high heat.
3. Add the chicken breasts to the skillet and cook for 6-7 minutes per side until cooked through and golden brown.
4. Remove the chicken breasts from the skillet and let them rest for a few minutes before slicing.
5. In a large salad bowl, combine the chopped romaine lettuce and grated Parmesan cheese.
6. Add the sliced chicken breasts to the salad bowl.
7. Drizzle the Caesar dressing over the salad and toss gently to coat.
8. Divide the salad between two plates.
9. If desired, sprinkle keto-friendly croutons over the salad for added texture and flavor.

10. Serve immediately and enjoy your classic and delicious keto chicken Caesar salad!

Nutritional Info (per serving):
Calories: 378 | Total Fat: 24g | Saturated Fat: 6g | Cholesterol: 109mg | Sodium: 683mg | Total Carbohydrates: 5g | Dietary Fiber: 2g | Sugars: 1g | Protein: 33g

Recipe Name:____________________

Date: / /

Time:____

Rating: ☆☆☆☆☆

S/N	Ingredients	Adjustment

Cooking Experience: ______________________________

____

____

____

Notes:_____________________________________

____

____

____

____

____

____

____

Keto Salmon and Asparagus Foil Packets

Prep Time: 10 minutes

Cooking Time: 20 minutes

Servings: 2

Ingredients:

- 2 salmon fillets (6 ounces each)
- 1 bunch asparagus, trimmed
- 2 tablespoons melted butter or olive oil
- 2 cloves garlic, minced
- 1 teaspoon lemon zest
- 1 tablespoon fresh lemon juice
- Salt and pepper to taste
- Fresh dill for garnish (optional)

Method of Preparation:

1. Preheat your oven to 375°F (190°C).
2. Cut two large pieces of aluminum foil and place them on a flat surface.
3. Divide the asparagus spears between the foil pieces, placing them in the center.
4. Season the salmon fillets with salt and pepper on both sides, then place one fillet on top of the asparagus on each foil piece.
5. In a small bowl, whisk together the melted butter or olive oil, minced garlic, lemon zest, and fresh lemon juice.
6. Drizzle the lemon butter mixture over the salmon and asparagus.

7. Fold the edges of the foil over the salmon and asparagus to create a packet, sealing tightly.
8. Place the foil packets on a baking sheet and bake in the preheated oven for 15-20 minutes until the salmon is cooked through and the asparagus is tender.
9. Carefully open the foil packets and transfer the salmon and asparagus to serving plates.
10. Garnish with fresh dill if desired.
11. Serve hot and enjoy your flavorful and nutritious keto salmon and asparagus foil packets!

Nutritional Info (per serving):
Calories: 347 | Total Fat: 22g | Saturated Fat: 7g | Cholesterol: 108mg | Sodium: 157mg | Total Carbohydrates: 6g | Dietary Fiber: 3g | Sugars: 2g | Protein: 32g

Recipe Name:______________________________

Date: / /

Time:_____

Rating: ☆☆☆☆☆

S/N	Ingredients	Adjustment

Cooking Experience: ____

____

____

____

Notes:____

____

____

____

____

____

____

____

Keto Egg Salad Lettuce Wraps

Prep Time: 10 minutes

Cooking Time: 10 minutes

Servings: 2

Ingredients:

- 4 large eggs
- 1/4 cup mayonnaise (keto-friendly)
- 1 tablespoon Dijon mustard
- 2 tablespoons chopped celery
- 2 tablespoons chopped green onions
- Salt and pepper to taste
- 4 large lettuce leaves (such as butter lettuce or romaine)
- **Optional toppings:** sliced avocado, cooked bacon, cherry tomatoes

Method of Preparation:

1. Place the eggs in a saucepan and cover them with water. Bring to a boil over medium-high heat.
2. Once boiling, cover the saucepan with a lid, remove from heat, and let the eggs sit in the hot water for 10 minutes.
3. Drain the hot water and transfer the eggs to a bowl of ice water to cool.
4. Once cool, peel the eggs and chop them into small pieces.
5. In a mixing bowl, combine the chopped eggs, mayonnaise, Dijon mustard, chopped celery, and chopped green onions. Mix well to combine.
6. Season the egg salad with salt and pepper to taste.
7. Lay out the lettuce leaves on a clean work surface.
8. Spoon the egg salad onto the center of each lettuce leaf.

9. If desired, top the egg salad with sliced avocado, cooked bacon, or cherry tomatoes.
10. Roll up the lettuce leaves tightly to form wraps.
11. Secure the wraps with toothpicks if needed.
12. Serve immediately and enjoy your creamy and flavorful keto egg salad lettuce wraps!

Nutritional Info (per serving):
Calories: 293 | Total Fat: 25g | Saturated Fat: 5g | Cholesterol: 373mg | Sodium: 408mg | Total Carbohydrates: 2g | Dietary Fiber: 1g | Sugars: 1g | Protein: 14g

Recipe Name:______________________

Date: / /

Time:**____**

Rating: ☆☆☆☆☆

S/N	Ingredients	Adjustment

Cooking Experience: ______________________________

____

____

____

Notes:______________________________

____

____

____

____

____

____

____

Keto Caprese Salad with Grilled Chicken

Prep Time: 15 minutes
Cooking Time: 10 minutes
Servings: 2
Ingredients:

- 2 boneless, skinless chicken breasts
- 1 tablespoon olive oil
- Salt and pepper to taste
- 1 cup cherry tomatoes, halved
- 4 ounces fresh mozzarella cheese, sliced
- 1/4 cup fresh basil leaves
- 2 tablespoons balsamic glaze (keto-friendly)
- Salt and pepper to taste

Method of Preparation:

1. Preheat a grill or grill pan over medium-high heat.
2. Season the chicken breasts with salt and pepper on both sides.
3. Drizzle the olive oil over the chicken breasts.
4. Grill the chicken breasts for 4-5 minutes per side until cooked through and grill marks appear.
5. Remove the chicken breasts from the grill and let them rest for a few minutes before slicing.
6. In a large bowl, combine the halved cherry tomatoes, sliced fresh mozzarella cheese, and fresh basil leaves.
7. Drizzle the balsamic glaze over the salad and toss gently to coat.
8. Divide the salad between two plates.

9. Top each salad with sliced grilled chicken breasts.
10. Season with salt and pepper to taste.
11. Serve immediately and enjoy your delicious and satisfying keto Caprese salad with grilled chicken!

Nutritional Info (per serving):
Calories: 374 | Total Fat: 20g | Saturated Fat: 9g | Cholesterol: 110mg | Sodium: 379mg | Total Carbohydrates: 6g | Dietary Fiber: 1g | Sugars: 4g | Protein: 41g

Recipe Name:____________________________

Date: / / ***Time:***_____

Rating: ☆☆☆☆☆

S/N	Ingredients	Adjustment

Cooking Experience: ____________________________

____

____

____

Notes:____________________________________

____

____

____

____

____

____

____

Keto Taco Salad Bowl

Prep Time: 15 minutes
Cooking Time: 15 minutes
Servings: 2
Ingredients:

- 1 tablespoon olive oil
- 1/2 pound ground beef
- 1 teaspoon chili powder
- 1/2 teaspoon ground cumin
- 1/2 teaspoon paprika
- 1/4 teaspoon garlic powder
- Salt and pepper to taste
- 4 cups shredded lettuce
- 1/2 cup cherry tomatoes, halved
- 1/4 cup shredded cheddar cheese
- 1/4 cup diced avocado
- 2 tablespoons sour cream (keto-friendly)
- 2 tablespoons salsa (keto-friendly)
- Fresh cilantro for garnish (optional)

Method of Preparation:

1. Heat the olive oil in a skillet over medium heat.
2. Add the ground beef to the skillet and cook, breaking it apart with a spoon, until browned and cooked through.
3. Stir in the chili powder, ground cumin, paprika, garlic powder, salt, and pepper. Cook for an additional 2-3 minutes to allow the flavors to meld.
4. Remove the skillet from heat and set aside.

5. In a large bowl, assemble the taco salad by layering the shredded lettuce, cooked ground beef, cherry tomatoes, shredded cheddar cheese, and diced avocado.
6. Top the salad with dollops of sour cream and salsa.
7. Garnish with fresh cilantro if desired.
8. Serve immediately and enjoy your flavorful and satisfying keto taco salad bowl!

Nutritional Info (per serving):
Calories: 415 | Total Fat: 30g | Saturated Fat: 10g | Cholesterol: 87mg | Sodium: 231mg | Total Carbohydrates: 8g | Dietary Fiber: 4g | Sugars: 2g | Protein: 29g

Recipe Name:___________________________

Date: / / ***Time:***____

Rating: ☆☆☆☆☆

S/N	Ingredients	Adjustment

Cooking Experience: ______________________________

____

____

____

Notes:____

____

____

____

____

____

____

____

Keto Broccoli and Bacon Salad

Prep Time: 15 minutes

Cooking Time: 10 minutes

Servings: 2

Ingredients:

- 4 cups fresh broccoli florets
- 4 slices cooked bacon, chopped
- 1/4 cup chopped red onion
- 1/4 cup shredded cheddar cheese
- 2 tablespoons chopped almonds or pecans
- 1/4 cup keto-friendly mayonnaise
- 1 tablespoon apple cider vinegar
- 1 teaspoon keto-friendly sweetener (such as erythritol or stevia)
- Salt and pepper to taste

Method of Preparation:

1. Steam the broccoli florets until tender-crisp, about 3-4 minutes. Drain and rinse with cold water to stop the cooking process.
2. In a large bowl, combine the steamed broccoli florets, chopped bacon, chopped red onion, shredded cheddar cheese, and chopped almonds or pecans.
3. In a small bowl, whisk together the keto-friendly mayonnaise, apple cider vinegar, and keto-friendly sweetener until well combined.
4. Pour the dressing over the broccoli salad and toss gently to coat.
5. Season with salt and pepper to taste.
6. Serve immediately or refrigerate until ready to serve.

7. Enjoy your crunchy and flavorful keto broccoli and bacon salad as a delicious lunch option!

Nutritional Info (per serving):
Calories: 349 | Total Fat: 29g | Saturated Fat: 7g | Cholesterol: 35mg | Sodium: 421mg | Total Carbohydrates: 9g | Dietary Fiber: 4g | Sugars: 2g | Protein: 14g

Recipe Name:______________________

Date: / / ***Time:***____

Rating: ☆☆☆☆☆

S/N	Ingredients	Adjustment

Cooking Experience: ______________________________

____

____

____

Notes:______________________________

____

____

____

____

____

____

____

CHAPTER FOUR

Dinner Recipes

Keto Lemon Garlic Butter Salmon

Prep Time: 10 minutes
Cooking Time: 15 minutes
Servings: 2
Ingredients:

- 2 salmon fillets (6 ounces each)
- Salt and pepper to taste
- 2 tablespoons unsalted butter
- 2 cloves garlic, minced
- Zest of 1 lemon
- Juice of 1/2 lemon
- 1 tablespoon chopped fresh parsley

Method of Preparation:

1. Preheat your oven to 375°F (190°C). Line a baking sheet with parchment paper.
2. Season the salmon fillets with salt and pepper on both sides.
3. In a small saucepan, melt the butter over medium heat. Add the minced garlic and cook for 1-2 minutes until fragrant.
4. Remove the saucepan from heat and stir in the lemon zest and lemon juice.
5. Place the salmon fillets on the prepared baking sheet.
6. Brush the lemon garlic butter mixture over the tops of the salmon fillets, reserving some for serving.
7. Bake in the preheated oven for 12-15 minutes until the salmon is cooked through and flakes easily with a fork.

8. Remove from the oven and sprinkle with chopped fresh parsley.
9. Serve the salmon hot with the remaining lemon garlic butter drizzled on top.
10. Enjoy your succulent and flavorful keto lemon garlic butter salmon!

Nutritional Info (per serving):
Calories: 341 | Total Fat: 22g | Saturated Fat: 7g | Cholesterol: 104mg | Sodium: 91mg | Total Carbohydrates: 2g | Dietary Fiber: 0g | Sugars: 0g | Protein: 32g

Recipe Name:____________________

Date: / /

Time:**_____**

Rating: ☆☆☆☆☆

S/N	Ingredients	Adjustment

Cooking Experience: ______________________________

____

____

____

Notes:______________________________________

____

____

____

____

____

____

____

Keto Cauliflower Alfredo with Chicken

Prep Time: 10 minutes
Cooking Time: 20 minutes
Servings: 2
Ingredients:

- 2 boneless, skinless chicken breasts
- Salt and pepper to taste
- 1 tablespoon olive oil
- 4 cups cauliflower florets
- 2 cloves garlic, minced
- 1 cup chicken broth
- 1/2 cup heavy cream
- 1/4 cup grated Parmesan cheese
- 2 tablespoons unsalted butter
- 1 tablespoon chopped fresh parsley

Method of Preparation:

1. Season the chicken breasts with salt and pepper on both sides.
2. Heat the olive oil in a skillet over medium heat. Add the chicken breasts and cook for 4-5 minutes per side until golden brown and cooked through. Remove from the skillet and set aside.
3. In a large saucepan, bring water to a boil. Add the cauliflower florets and cook for 6-8 minutes until tender. Drain the cauliflower and set aside.
4. In the same skillet used for the chicken, add minced garlic and sauté for 1-2 minutes until fragrant.

5. Add the chicken broth to the skillet and bring to a simmer.
6. Transfer the cooked cauliflower to a blender. Pour the simmering chicken broth and garlic mixture over the cauliflower.
7. Add the heavy cream, grated Parmesan cheese, and unsalted butter to the blender.
8. Blend until smooth and creamy, adding more chicken broth or cream if needed to reach your desired consistency.
9. Season the cauliflower Alfredo sauce with salt and pepper to taste.
10. Slice the cooked chicken breasts and serve over a bed of cooked low-carb noodles or zucchini noodles.
11. Pour the cauliflower Alfredo sauce over the chicken.
12. Garnish with chopped fresh parsley before serving.
13. Enjoy your indulgent and satisfying keto cauliflower Alfredo with chicken!

Nutritional Info (per serving):
Calories: 476 | Total Fat: 32g | Saturated Fat: 17g | Cholesterol: 162mg | Sodium: 747mg | Total Carbohydrates: 8g | Dietary Fiber: 3g | Sugars: 3g | Protein: 39g

Recipe Name:_______________

Date: / /

Time:_____

Rating: ☆☆☆☆☆

S/N	Ingredients	Adjustment

Cooking Experience: _______________

____

____

____

Notes:_______________

____

____

____

____

____

____

____

Keto Beef and Broccoli Stir-Fry

Prep Time: 15 minutes

Cooking Time: 15 minutes

Servings: 2

Ingredients:

- 8 ounces flank steak, thinly sliced against the grain
- 2 tablespoons soy sauce or tamari (for gluten-free)
- 1 tablespoon sesame oil
- 2 cloves garlic, minced
- 1 teaspoon grated ginger
- 1 tablespoon olive oil
- 2 cups broccoli florets
- 1/2 cup sliced bell peppers (any color)
- Salt and pepper to taste
- Sesame seeds for garnish (optional)
- Sliced green onions for garnish (optional)

Method of Preparation:

1. In a bowl, marinate the thinly sliced flank steak with soy sauce (or tamari), sesame oil, minced garlic, and grated ginger. Set aside for 10-15 minutes.
2. Heat olive oil in a large skillet or wok over medium-high heat.
3. Add the marinated flank steak to the skillet and cook for 2-3 minutes until browned.
4. Remove the steak from the skillet and set aside.
5. In the same skillet, add the broccoli florets and sliced bell peppers. Stir-fry for 4-5 minutes until the vegetables are tender-crisp.

6. Return the cooked steak to the skillet and toss with the vegetables.
7. Season with salt and pepper to taste.
8. Continue to stir-fry for another 1-2 minutes until everything is heated through.
9. Remove from heat and garnish with sesame seeds and sliced green onions if desired.
10. Serve hot and enjoy your delicious and nutritious keto beef and broccoli stir-fry!

Nutritional Info (per serving):
Calories: 303 | Total Fat: 19g | Saturated Fat: 5g | Cholesterol: 62mg | Sodium: 873mg | Total Carbohydrates: 9g | Dietary Fiber: 3g | Sugars: 3g | Protein: 25g

Recipe Name:__________________________

Date: / /   ***Time:***_____

Rating: ☆☆☆☆☆

S/N	Ingredients	Adjustment

Cooking Experience: ______________________________

Notes:____

Keto Spaghetti Squash with Meatballs

Prep Time: 15 minutes

Cooking Time: 1 hour

Servings: 2

Ingredients:

For the Meatballs:

- 1/2-pound ground beef
- 1/4 cup grated Parmesan cheese
- 1/4 cup almond flour
- 1 egg
- 2 cloves garlic, minced
- 1 tablespoon chopped fresh parsley
- Salt and pepper to taste

For the Spaghetti Squash:

- 1 medium spaghetti squash
- 1 tablespoon olive oil
- Salt and pepper to taste
- Keto-friendly marinara sauce

Method of Preparation:

1. Preheat your oven to 375°F (190°C).
2. Cut the spaghetti squash in half lengthwise and scoop out the seeds.
3. Brush the cut sides of the spaghetti squash with olive oil and season with salt and pepper.
4. Place the spaghetti squash halves cut-side down on a baking sheet lined with parchment paper.

5. Bake in the preheated oven for 45-50 minutes until the squash is tender and easily pierced with a fork.
6. While the spaghetti squash is baking, prepare the meatballs. In a bowl, combine the ground beef, grated Parmesan cheese, almond flour, egg, minced garlic, chopped fresh parsley, salt, and pepper. Mix until well combined.
7. Roll the mixture into meatballs, about 1 inch in diameter.
8. Heat a skillet over medium heat and add a little olive oil. Cook the meatballs for 8-10 minutes, turning occasionally, until browned on all sides and cooked through.
9. Once the spaghetti squash is done baking, use a fork to scrape the flesh into spaghetti-like strands.
10. Serve the spaghetti squash topped with keto-friendly marinara sauce and meatballs.
11. Garnish with additional grated Parmesan cheese and chopped fresh parsley if desired.
12. Enjoy your hearty and satisfying keto spaghetti squash with meatballs!

Nutritional Info (per serving):
Calories: 418 | Total Fat: 26g | Saturated Fat: 8g | Cholesterol: 134mg | Sodium: 355mg | Total Carbohydrates: 20g | Dietary Fiber: 5g | Sugars: 7g | Protein: 28g

Recipe Name:______________________________

Date: / / ***Time:*____**

Rating: ☆☆☆☆☆

S/N	Ingredients	Adjustment

Cooking Experience: ______________________________

____

____

____

Notes:______________________________

____

____

____

____

____

____

____

Keto Chicken Alfredo Zucchini Boats

Prep Time: 20 minutes

Cooking Time: 25 minutes

Servings: 2

Ingredients:

- 2 medium zucchinis
- 1 tablespoon olive oil
- Salt and pepper to taste
- 2 boneless, skinless chicken breasts, diced
- 2 cloves garlic, minced
- 1 cup heavy cream
- 1/2 cup grated Parmesan cheese
- 1 tablespoon chopped fresh parsley
- **Optional:** keto-friendly Italian seasoning blend

Method of Preparation:

1. Preheat your oven to 400°F (200°C).
2. Cut the zucchinis in half lengthwise. Use a spoon to scoop out the flesh from the center, leaving about 1/4 inch around the edges to form boats. Reserve the zucchini flesh for later use.
3. Place the zucchini boats on a baking sheet lined with parchment paper. Brush the insides with olive oil and season with salt and pepper.
4. In a skillet, heat olive oil over medium heat. Add the diced chicken breasts and minced garlic. Cook until the chicken is browned and cooked through.
5. Meanwhile, chop the reserved zucchini flesh into small pieces.

6. Add the chopped zucchini to the skillet with the cooked chicken. Cook for another 2-3 minutes until the zucchini is tender.
7. Reduce the heat to low and pour in the heavy cream. Stir in the grated Parmesan cheese until melted and well combined.
8. Season the mixture with salt, pepper, and optional Italian seasoning to taste. Simmer for a few minutes until the sauce thickens slightly.
9. Spoon the chicken Alfredo mixture into the zucchini boats, filling them evenly.
10. Place the filled zucchini boats back on the baking sheet and bake in the preheated oven for 15 minutes.
11. Garnish with chopped fresh parsley before serving.
12. Enjoy your creamy and delicious keto chicken Alfredo zucchini boats!

Nutritional Info (per serving):
Calories: 470 | Total Fat: 33g | Saturated Fat: 18g | Cholesterol: 181mg | Sodium: 539mg | Total Carbohydrates: 8g | Dietary Fiber: 2g | Sugars: 4g | Protein: 35g

Recipe Name:____________________

Date: / /   ***Time:***_____

Rating: ☆☆☆☆☆

S/N	Ingredients	Adjustment

Cooking Experience: ______________________________

____

____

____

Notes:______________________________

____

____

____

____

____

____

____

Keto Shrimp Stir-Fry with Cauliflower Rice

Prep Time: 15 minutes
Cooking Time: 15 minutes
Servings: 2
Ingredients:

- 1 pound large shrimp, peeled and deveined
- 1 tablespoon olive oil
- 2 cloves garlic, minced
- 1 teaspoon grated ginger
- 1 cup broccoli florets
- 1/2 cup sliced bell peppers (any color)
- 1/2 cup sliced mushrooms
- 1/4 cup sliced green onions
- 2 cups cauliflower rice
- 2 tablespoons soy sauce or tamari (for gluten-free)
- 1 tablespoon sesame oil
- Sesame seeds for garnish (optional)
- Sliced green onions for garnish (optional)

Method of Preparation:

1. Heat olive oil in a large skillet or wok over medium-high heat.
2. Add minced garlic and grated ginger to the skillet and sauté for 1 minute until fragrant.
3. Add the shrimp to the skillet and cook for 2-3 minutes until pink and opaque. Remove the shrimp from the skillet and set aside.

4. In the same skillet, add broccoli florets, sliced bell peppers, and sliced mushrooms. Stir-fry for 4-5 minutes until the vegetables are tender-crisp.
5. Push the vegetables to one side of the skillet and add cauliflower rice to the empty space. Cook for 2-3 minutes until heated through.
6. Return the cooked shrimp to the skillet and toss with the vegetables and cauliflower rice.
7. Drizzle soy sauce or tamari and sesame oil over the shrimp stir-fry. Stir well to combine.
8. Cook for another 1-2 minutes until everything is heated through and well coated with the sauce.
9. Remove from heat and garnish with sesame seeds and sliced green onions if desired.
10. Serve hot and enjoy your flavorful and nutritious keto shrimp stir-fry with cauliflower rice!

Nutritional Info (per serving):
Calories: 317 | Total Fat: 12g | Saturated Fat: 2g | Cholesterol: 344mg | Sodium: 1182mg | Total Carbohydrates: 14g | Dietary Fiber: 5g | Sugars: 5g | Protein: 40g

Recipe Name:____________________

Date: / /   ***Time:***_____

Rating: ☆☆☆☆☆

S/N	Ingredients	Adjustment

Cooking Experience: ____________________

____

____

____

Notes:____________________

____

____

____

____

____

____

____

Keto Beef and Vegetable Stir-Fry

Prep Time: 15 minutes

Cooking Time: 15 minutes

Servings: 2

Ingredients:

- 8 ounces beef sirloin, thinly sliced
- 2 tablespoons soy sauce or tamari (for gluten-free)
- 1 tablespoon olive oil
- 2 cloves garlic, minced
- 1 teaspoon grated ginger
- 1 cup broccoli florets
- 1/2 cup sliced bell peppers (any color)
- 1/2 cup sliced mushrooms
- 1/4 cup sliced carrots
- 1/4 cup sliced green onions
- Salt and pepper to taste
- Sesame seeds for garnish (optional)

Method of Preparation:

1. In a bowl, marinate the thinly sliced beef sirloin with soy sauce (or tamari). Set aside for 10-15 minutes.
2. Heat olive oil in a large skillet or wok over medium-high heat.
3. Add minced garlic and grated ginger to the skillet and sauté for 1 minute until fragrant.
4. Add the marinated beef sirloin to the skillet and cook for 2-3 minutes until browned. Remove the beef from the skillet and set aside.

5. In the same skillet, add broccoli florets, sliced bell peppers, sliced mushrooms, and sliced carrots. Stir-fry for 4-5 minutes until the vegetables are tender-crisp.
6. Return the cooked beef to the skillet and toss with the vegetables.
7. Season with salt and pepper to taste.
8. Cook for another 1-2 minutes until everything is heated through.
9. Remove from heat and garnish with sesame seeds if desired.
10. Serve hot and enjoy your delicious and nutritious keto beef and vegetable stir-fry!

Nutritional Info (per serving):
Calories: 298 | Total Fat: 17g | Saturated Fat: 4g | Cholesterol: 66mg | Sodium: 937mg | Total Carbohydrates: 10g | Dietary Fiber: 3g | Sugars: 4g | Protein: 25g

Recipe Name:________________________

Date: / /   ***Time:*****____**

Rating: ☆ ☆ ☆ ☆ ☆

S/N	Ingredients	Adjustment

Cooking Experience: ______________________________

____

____

____

Notes:______________________________________

____

____

____

____

____

____

____

Keto Zucchini Lasagna

Prep Time: 20 minutes
Cooking Time: 45 minutes
Servings: 2
Ingredients:

- 2 medium zucchinis, sliced lengthwise into thin strips
- 1 cup marinara sauce (keto-friendly)
- 8 ounces ground beef
- 1/2 cup ricotta cheese
- 1/4 cup grated Parmesan cheese
- 1/2 cup shredded mozzarella cheese
- 1 tablespoon chopped fresh basil
- Salt and pepper to taste

Method of Preparation:

1. Preheat your oven to 375°F (190°C).
2. In a skillet, cook the ground beef over medium heat until browned. Drain excess fat.
3. Stir in the marinara sauce and simmer for 5 minutes.
4. In a bowl, combine the ricotta cheese, grated Parmesan cheese, chopped fresh basil, salt, and pepper.
5. Spread a thin layer of the meat sauce in the bottom of a baking dish.
6. Arrange a layer of zucchini slices on top of the meat sauce.
7. Spread a layer of the ricotta cheese mixture over the zucchini slices.
8. Repeat the layers until all ingredients are used, finishing with a layer of meat sauce on top.
9. Sprinkle the shredded mozzarella cheese evenly over the top layer.

10. Cover the baking dish with foil and bake in the preheated oven for 30 minutes.
11. Remove the foil and bake for an additional 15 minutes until the cheese is melted and bubbly.
12. Let the lasagna cool for a few minutes before slicing and serving.
13. Enjoy your comforting and satisfying keto zucchini lasagna!

Nutritional Info (per serving):

Calories: 433 | Total Fat: 28g | Saturated Fat: 14g | Cholesterol: 111mg | Sodium: 933mg | Total Carbohydrates: 11g | Dietary Fiber: 3g | Sugars: 6g | Protein: 34g

Recipe Name:________________________

Date: / /

Time: ____

Rating: ☆☆☆☆☆

S/N	Ingredients	Adjustment

Cooking Experience: ________________________________

____

____

____

Notes: ____

____

____

____

____

____

____

____

Keto Spinach and Feta Stuffed Chicken Breast

Prep Time: 15 minutes

Cooking Time: 25 minutes

Servings: 2

Ingredients:

- 2 boneless, skinless chicken breasts
- Salt and pepper to taste
- 1 cup fresh spinach leaves
- 1/4 cup crumbled feta cheese
- 2 cloves garlic, minced
- 1 tablespoon olive oil
- 1/2 teaspoon dried oregano
- 1/2 teaspoon dried basil
- Toothpicks

Method of Preparation:

1. Preheat your oven to 375°F (190°C). Grease a baking dish with olive oil or line it with parchment paper.
2. Using a sharp knife, carefully slice each chicken breast horizontally to create a pocket without cutting all the way through.
3. Season the inside of each chicken breast with salt and pepper.
4. In a small skillet, heat olive oil over medium heat. Add minced garlic and sauté for 1-2 minutes until fragrant.
5. Add fresh spinach leaves to the skillet and cook for 2-3 minutes until wilted.

6. Remove the skillet from heat and stir in crumbled feta cheese, dried oregano, and dried basil.
7. Stuff each chicken breast with the spinach and feta mixture.
8. Secure the openings of the chicken breasts with toothpicks to prevent the filling from falling out.
9. Place the stuffed chicken breasts in the prepared baking dish.
10. Bake in the preheated oven for 20-25 minutes until the chicken is cooked through and no longer pink in the center.
11. Remove the toothpicks before serving.
12. Serve hot and enjoy your flavorful and nutritious keto spinach and feta stuffed chicken breasts!

Nutritional Info (per serving):
Calories: 290 | Total Fat: 15g | Saturated Fat: 5g | Cholesterol: 102mg | Sodium: 325mg | Total Carbohydrates: 2g | Dietary Fiber: 1g | Sugars: 0g | Protein: 36g

Recipe Name:______________________________

Date: / / ***Time:***_____

Rating: ☆☆☆☆☆

S/N	Ingredients	Adjustment

Cooking Experience: ______________________________

Notes:____________________________________

Keto Pork Tenderloin with Garlic-Herb Butter

Prep Time: 10 minutes
Cooking Time: 25 minutes
Servings: 2
Ingredients:

- 1 pork tenderloin (about 1 pound)
- Salt and pepper to taste
- 2 tablespoons olive oil
- 2 tablespoons unsalted butter, softened
- 2 cloves garlic, minced
- 1 tablespoon chopped fresh parsley
- 1 teaspoon chopped fresh thyme
- 1 teaspoon chopped fresh rosemary

Method of Preparation:

1. Preheat your oven to 375°F (190°C).
2. Season the pork tenderloin with salt and pepper on all sides.
3. Heat olive oil in an oven-safe skillet over medium-high heat.
4. Add the seasoned pork tenderloin to the skillet and sear for 2-3 minutes on each side until browned.
5. In a small bowl, combine softened butter, minced garlic, chopped fresh parsley, chopped fresh thyme, and chopped fresh rosemary to make the garlic-herb butter.
6. Spread the garlic-herb butter over the top of the seared pork tenderloin.
7. Transfer the skillet to the preheated oven and roast for 20-25 minutes until the pork reaches an internal temperature of 145°F (63°C) for medium doneness.

8. Remove the pork tenderloin from the oven and let it rest for 5 minutes before slicing.
9. Slice the pork tenderloin into medallions and serve hot.
10. Enjoy your succulent and flavorful keto pork tenderloin with garlic-herb butter!

Nutritional Info (per serving):
Calories: 384 | Total Fat: 27g | Saturated Fat: 9g | Cholesterol: 130mg | Sodium: 176mg | Total Carbohydrates: 1g | Dietary Fiber: 0g | Sugars: 0g | Protein: 35g

Recipe Name:___________________________

Date: / /

Time:_____

Rating: ☆☆☆☆☆

S/N	Ingredients	Adjustment

Cooking Experience: ___________________________

____

____

____

Notes:___________________________

____

____

____

____

____

____

____

CHAPTER FIVE

Dessert Recipes

Keto Chocolate Avocado Mousse

Prep Time: 10 minutes

Cooking Time: 0 minutes

Servings: 2

Ingredients:

- 1 ripe avocado, peeled and pitted
- 1/4 cup unsweetened cocoa powder
- 1/4 cup keto-friendly sweetener (such as erythritol or stevia)
- 1/4 cup unsweetened almond milk (or coconut milk)
- 1 teaspoon vanilla extract
- Pinch of salt
- **Optional toppings:** whipped cream, shaved dark chocolate, berries

Method of Preparation:

1. In a blender or food processor, combine the ripe avocado, unsweetened cocoa powder, keto-friendly sweetener, unsweetened almond milk, vanilla extract, and a pinch of salt.
2. Blend until smooth and creamy, scraping down the sides of the blender or food processor as needed.
3. Taste and adjust sweetness if necessary by adding more sweetener.
4. Divide the chocolate avocado mousse into serving glasses or bowls.
5. Refrigerate for at least 30 minutes to allow the mousse to set.

6. Before serving, top with whipped cream, shaved dark chocolate, or berries if desired.
7. Serve chilled and enjoy your indulgent yet healthy keto chocolate avocado mousse!

Nutritional Info (per serving):
Calories: 194 | Total Fat: 15g | Saturated Fat: 3g | Cholesterol: 0mg | Sodium: 10mg | Total Carbohydrates: 15g | Dietary Fiber: 9g | Sugars: 1g | Protein: 4g

Recipe Name:________________________

Date: / / ***Time:***_____

Rating: ☆☆☆☆☆

S/N	Ingredients	Adjustment

Cooking Experience: ______________________________

____

____

____

Notes:______________________________

____

____

____

____

____

____

____

Keto Coconut Almond Fat Bombs

Prep Time: 10 minutes

Cooking Time: 0 minutes

Servings: 8

Ingredients:

- 1/2 cup coconut oil, melted
- 1/4 cup unsweetened shredded coconut
- 1/4 cup almond flour
- 2 tablespoons keto-friendly sweetener (such as erythritol or stevia)
- 1/2 teaspoon vanilla extract
- Pinch of salt
- **Optional:** dark chocolate chips, chopped nuts

Method of Preparation:

1. In a mixing bowl, combine melted coconut oil, unsweetened shredded coconut, almond flour, keto-friendly sweetener, vanilla extract, and a pinch of salt.
2. Stir until well combined and the mixture resembles a thick paste.
3. If desired, fold in dark chocolate chips or chopped nuts for added texture and flavor.
4. Line a mini muffin tin with paper liners.
5. Spoon the coconut almond mixture into the muffin tin, filling each cavity about halfway full.
6. Place the muffin tin in the freezer and freeze for 30 minutes to set the fat bombs.
7. Once set, remove the fat bombs from the muffin tin and store them in an airtight container in the refrigerator.

8. Enjoy these delicious and satisfying keto coconut almond fat bombs as a guilt-free dessert or snack!

Nutritional Info (per serving - 1 fat bomb):
Calories: 123 | Total Fat: 13g | Saturated Fat: 10g | Cholesterol: 0mg | Sodium: 16mg | Total Carbohydrates: 2g | Dietary Fiber: 1g | Sugars: 0g | Protein: 1g

Recipe Name:________________________

Date: / / ***Time:***_____

Rating: ☆☆☆☆☆

S/N	Ingredients	Adjustment

Cooking Experience: ______________________________

____

____

____

Notes:______________________________

____

____

____

____

____

____

____

Keto Berry Chia Seed Pudding

Prep Time: 5 minutes
Cooking Time: 0 minutes
Chilling Time: 4 hours
Servings: 2
Ingredients:

- 1 cup unsweetened almond milk (or coconut milk)
- 1/4 cup chia seeds
- 2 tablespoons keto-friendly sweetener (such as erythritol or stevia)
- 1/2 teaspoon vanilla extract
- 1/2 cup mixed berries (such as strawberries, blueberries, raspberries)

Method of Preparation:

1. In a mixing bowl, whisk together unsweetened almond milk, chia seeds, keto-friendly sweetener, and vanilla extract.
2. Let the mixture sit for 5 minutes, then whisk again to break up any clumps of chia seeds.
3. Cover the bowl and refrigerate for at least 4 hours or overnight, allowing the chia seeds to absorb the liquid and thicken into a pudding-like consistency.
4. Before serving, stir the chia seed pudding to evenly distribute the seeds.
5. Divide the pudding into serving glasses or bowls.
6. Top with mixed berries just before serving.
7. Enjoy your refreshing and nutritious keto berry chia seed pudding as a delightful dessert or snack!

Nutritional Info (per serving):
Calories: 140 | Total Fat: 8g | Saturated Fat: 0.5g | Cholesterol: 0mg | Sodium: 80mg | Total Carbohydrates: 15g | Dietary Fiber: 10g | Sugars: 2g | Protein: 4g

Recipe Name:________________________

***Date:* / /** ***Time:*____**

Rating: ☆☆☆☆☆

S/N	Ingredients	Adjustment

Cooking Experience: ______________________________

Notes:____________________________________

Keto Peanut Butter Chocolate Fat Bombs

Prep Time: 10 minutes
Cooking Time: 0 minutes
Chilling Time: 1 hour
Servings: 8
Ingredients:

- 1/2 cup natural peanut butter (unsweetened)
- 1/4 cup coconut oil, melted
- 2 tablespoons unsweetened cocoa powder
- 2 tablespoons keto-friendly sweetener (such as erythritol or stevia)
- 1/2 teaspoon vanilla extract
- Pinch of salt

Method of Preparation:

1. In a mixing bowl, combine natural peanut butter, melted coconut oil, unsweetened cocoa powder, keto-friendly sweetener, vanilla extract, and a pinch of salt.
2. Stir until all ingredients are well combined and the mixture is smooth.
3. Line a mini muffin tin with paper liners.
4. Spoon the peanut butter chocolate mixture into the muffin tin, filling each cavity about halfway full.
5. Place the muffin tin in the freezer and freeze for at least 1 hour to set the fat bombs.
6. Once set, remove the fat bombs from the muffin tin and store them in an airtight container in the refrigerator.
7. Enjoy these decadent keto peanut butter chocolate fat bombs as a satisfying dessert or snack!

Nutritional Info (per serving - 1 fat bomb):
Calories: 157 | Total Fat: 14g | Saturated Fat: 7g | Cholesterol: 0mg | Sodium: 54mg | Total Carbohydrates: 5g | Dietary Fiber: 2g | Sugars: 1g | Protein: 4g

Recipe Name:___________________________

Date: / / ***Time:***_____

Rating: ☆☆☆☆☆

S/N	Ingredients	Adjustment

Cooking Experience: ______________________________

____

____

____

Notes:____

____

____

____

____

____

____

____

Keto Lemon Coconut Bliss Balls

Prep Time: 15 minutes

Cooking Time: 0 minutes

Chilling Time: 30 minutes

Servings: 12

Ingredients:

- 1 cup unsweetened shredded coconut
- 1/4 cup almond flour
- 2 tablespoons keto-friendly sweetener (such as erythritol or stevia)
- Zest of 1 lemon
- 2 tablespoons lemon juice
- 2 tablespoons coconut oil, melted
- 1/2 teaspoon vanilla extract
- Pinch of salt

Method of Preparation:

1. In a food processor, combine unsweetened shredded coconut, almond flour, keto-friendly sweetener, lemon zest, lemon juice, melted coconut oil, vanilla extract, and a pinch of salt.
2. Pulse until the mixture comes together and forms a sticky dough.
3. Scoop out tablespoon-sized portions of the dough and roll them into balls using your hands.
4. Place the lemon coconut bliss balls on a baking sheet lined with parchment paper.
5. Refrigerate for at least 30 minutes to allow the balls to firm up.

6. Once chilled, store the bliss balls in an airtight container in the refrigerator until ready to serve.
7. Enjoy these refreshing and satisfying keto lemon coconut bliss balls as a delightful dessert or snack!

Nutritional Info (per serving - 1 bliss ball):
Calories: 81 | Total Fat: 8g | Saturated Fat: 6g | Cholesterol: 0mg | Sodium: 11mg | Total Carbohydrates: 2g | Dietary Fiber: 1g | Sugars: 0g | Protein: 1g

Recipe Name:______________________________

Date: / / ***Time:***_____

Rating: ☆☆☆☆☆

S/N	Ingredients	Adjustment

Cooking Experience: ______________________________

____

____

____

Notes:____________________________________

____

____

____

____

____

____

____

Keto Vanilla Almond Fat Bombs

Prep Time: 10 minutes

Cooking Time: 0 minutes

Chilling Time: 1 hour

Servings: 8

Ingredients:

- 1/2 cup almond butter (unsweetened)
- 1/4 cup coconut oil, melted
- 2 tablespoons almond flour
- 2 tablespoons keto-friendly sweetener (such as erythritol or stevia)
- 1 teaspoon vanilla extract
- Pinch of salt

Method of Preparation:

1. In a mixing bowl, combine almond butter, melted coconut oil, almond flour, keto-friendly sweetener, vanilla extract, and a pinch of salt.
2. Stir until all ingredients are well combined and the mixture is smooth.
3. Line a mini muffin tin with paper liners.
4. Spoon the almond mixture into the muffin tin, filling each cavity about halfway full.
5. Place the muffin tin in the freezer and freeze for at least 1 hour to set the fat bombs.
6. Once set, remove the fat bombs from the muffin tin and store them in an airtight container in the refrigerator.
7. Enjoy these delicious and satisfying keto vanilla almond fat bombs as a guilt-free dessert or snack!

Nutritional Info (per serving - 1 fat bomb):
Calories: 141 | Total Fat: 14g | Saturated Fat: 6g | Cholesterol: 0mg | Sodium: 34mg | Total Carbohydrates: 3g | Dietary Fiber: 1g | Sugars: 1g | Protein: 3g

Recipe Name:_______________________________

Date:* / /** ***Time:_____

Rating: ☆☆☆☆☆

S/N	Ingredients	Adjustment

Cooking Experience: ________________________________

____

____

____

Notes:______________________________________

____

____

____

____

____

____

____

Keto Chocolate Peanut Butter Cups

Prep Time: 15 minutes
Cooking Time: 0 minutes
Chilling Time: 1 hour
Servings: 12
Ingredients:

- 1/2 cup sugar-free chocolate chips
- 2 tablespoons coconut oil
- 1/4 cup natural peanut butter (unsweetened)
- 1 tablespoon keto-friendly sweetener (such as erythritol or stevia)
- Pinch of salt

Method of Preparation:

1. In a microwave-safe bowl, combine sugar-free chocolate chips and coconut oil.
2. Microwave in 30-second intervals, stirring between each interval, until the chocolate chips are melted and smooth.
3. In a separate bowl, mix together natural peanut butter, keto-friendly sweetener, and a pinch of salt until well combined.
4. Line a mini muffin tin with paper liners.
5. Spoon a small amount of melted chocolate mixture into each paper liner, spreading it to cover the bottom.
6. Place a small dollop of peanut butter mixture on top of the chocolate layer in each paper liner.
7. Cover the peanut butter layer with the remaining melted chocolate mixture.
8. Tap the muffin tin gently on the countertop to even out the chocolate layer.

9. Place the muffin tin in the freezer and freeze for at least 1 hour to set the peanut butter cups.
10. Once set, remove the peanut butter cups from the muffin tin and store them in an airtight container in the refrigerator.
11. Enjoy these decadent keto chocolate peanut butter cups as a delicious and satisfying dessert!

Nutritional Info (per serving - 1 peanut butter cup):
Calories: 86 | Total Fat: 8g | Saturated Fat: 4g | Cholesterol: 0mg | Sodium: 15mg | Total Carbohydrates: 3g | Dietary Fiber: 2g | Sugars: 0g | Protein: 2g

Recipe Name:______________________

Date: / / ***Time:***____

Rating: ☆☆☆☆☆

S/N	Ingredients	Adjustment

Cooking Experience: ______________________

____

____

____

Notes:______________________

____

____

____

____

____

____

____

Keto Coconut Flour Blueberry Muffins

Prep Time: 10 minutes
Cooking Time: 25 minutes
Servings: 6
Ingredients:

- 1/2 cup coconut flour
- 1/4 cup keto-friendly sweetener (such as erythritol or stevia)
- 1/2 teaspoon baking powder
- Pinch of salt
- 4 large eggs
- 1/4 cup coconut oil, melted
- 1/4 cup unsweetened almond milk (or coconut milk)
- 1 teaspoon vanilla extract
- 1/2 cup fresh blueberries

Method of Preparation:

1. Preheat your oven to 350°F (175°C). Line a muffin tin with paper liners or grease it with coconut oil.
2. In a mixing bowl, combine coconut flour, keto-friendly sweetener, baking powder, and a pinch of salt.
3. In a separate bowl, whisk together eggs, melted coconut oil, unsweetened almond milk, and vanilla extract until well combined.
4. Pour the wet ingredients into the dry ingredients and mix until a smooth batter forms.
5. Gently fold in fresh blueberries.
6. Divide the batter evenly among the muffin cups, filling each about 3/4 full.

7. Bake in the preheated oven for 20-25 minutes, or until the muffins are golden brown and a toothpick inserted into the center comes out clean.
8. Allow the muffins to cool in the tin for 5 minutes, then transfer them to a wire rack to cool completely.
9. Serve and enjoy these fluffy and flavorful keto coconut flour blueberry muffins as a delightful dessert or snack!

Nutritional Info (per serving - 1 muffin):
Calories: 149 | Total Fat: 12g | Saturated Fat: 9g | Cholesterol: 124mg | Sodium: 50mg | Total Carbohydrates: 6g | Dietary Fiber: 3g | Sugars: 1g | Protein: 5g

Recipe Name:______________________

Date: / / ***Time:***____

Rating: ☆☆☆☆☆

S/N	Ingredients	Adjustment

Cooking Experience: ______________________________

____

____

____

Notes:______________________________________

____

____

____

____

____

____

____

Keto Cheesecake Bites with Raspberry Swirl

Prep Time: 15 minutes

Cooking Time: 20 minutes

Chilling Time: 2 hours

Servings: 12

Ingredients:

- 8 ounces cream cheese, softened
- 1/4 cup keto-friendly sweetener (such as erythritol or stevia)
- 1 large egg
- 1 teaspoon vanilla extract
- 1/4 cup fresh raspberries
- 1 tablespoon keto-friendly sweetener (for raspberry swirl)

Method of Preparation:

1. Preheat your oven to 350°F (175°C). Line a muffin tin with paper liners.
2. In a mixing bowl, beat the softened cream cheese until smooth.
3. Add the keto-friendly sweetener, egg, and vanilla extract to the cream cheese. Beat until well combined and creamy.
4. In a separate bowl, mash the fresh raspberries with a fork until smooth. Stir in the additional tablespoon of keto-friendly sweetener.
5. Spoon the cream cheese mixture into the prepared muffin tin, filling each cup about halfway.
6. Add a small dollop of the raspberry mixture on top of the cream cheese mixture in each cup.
7. Use a toothpick to gently swirl the raspberry mixture into the cream cheese mixture, creating a marbled effect.

8. Bake in the preheated oven for 18-20 minutes, or until the cheesecake bites are set and slightly golden around the edges.
9. Remove from the oven and let the cheesecake bites cool in the muffin tin for 10 minutes.
10. Transfer the cheesecake bites to a wire rack to cool completely, then refrigerate for at least 2 hours before serving.
11. Enjoy these decadent keto cheesecake bites with raspberry swirl as a delightful dessert or snack!

Nutritional Info (per serving - 1 cheesecake bite):
Calories: 91 | Total Fat: 8g | Saturated Fat: 5g | Cholesterol: 39mg | Sodium: 70mg | Total Carbohydrates: 2g | Dietary Fiber: 0g | Sugars: 1g | Protein: 2g

Recipe Name:______________________

Date: / / ***Time:***_____

Rating: ☆☆☆☆☆

S/N	Ingredients	Adjustment

Cooking Experience: ______________________________

____

____

____

Notes:____________________________________

____

____

____

____

____

____

____

Keto Pumpkin Spice Fat Bombs

Prep Time: 10 minutes

Cooking Time: 0 minutes

Chilling Time: 1 hour

Servings: 8

Ingredients:

- 1/2 cup pumpkin puree (unsweetened)
- 1/4 cup coconut oil, melted
- 2 tablespoons almond flour
- 2 tablespoons keto-friendly sweetener (such as erythritol or stevia)
- 1/2 teaspoon pumpkin pie spice
- Pinch of salt

Method of Preparation:

1. In a mixing bowl, combine pumpkin puree, melted coconut oil, almond flour, keto-friendly sweetener, pumpkin pie spice, and a pinch of salt.
2. Stir until all ingredients are well combined and the mixture is smooth.
3. Line a mini muffin tin with paper liners.
4. Spoon the pumpkin spice mixture into the muffin tin, filling each cavity about halfway full.
5. Place the muffin tin in the freezer and freeze for at least 1 hour to set the fat bombs.
6. Once set, remove the fat bombs from the muffin tin and store them in an airtight container in the refrigerator.
7. Enjoy these festive and flavorful keto pumpkin spice fat bombs as a guilt-free dessert or snack!

Nutritional Info (per serving - 1 fat bomb):
Calories: 78 | Total Fat: 7g | Saturated Fat: 6g | Cholesterol: 0mg | Sodium: 7mg | Total Carbohydrates: 3g | Dietary Fiber: 1g | Sugars: 1g | Protein: 1g

Recipe Name:________________________

Date: / /

Time:_____

Rating: ☆☆☆☆☆

S/N	Ingredients	Adjustment

Cooking Experience: ______________________________________

Notes:____

CHAPTER SIX

Juicing Recipes

Green Keto Energizer Juice

Prep Time: 10 minutes

Cooking Time: 0 minutes

Servings: 1

Ingredients:

- 1 cup spinach leaves
- 1/2 cucumber, peeled
- 1/2 avocado, peeled and pitted
- 1/2 lemon, peeled
- 1 tablespoon fresh ginger, peeled
- 1 cup unsweetened almond milk (or coconut milk)
- 1/2 cup cold water
- Ice cubes (optional)

Method of Preparation:

1. Wash the spinach leaves thoroughly and chop the cucumber into chunks.
2. In a blender, combine spinach leaves, cucumber chunks, peeled avocado, peeled lemon, peeled ginger, unsweetened almond milk, and cold water.
3. Blend on high speed until the ingredients are well combined and the mixture is smooth.
4. If desired, add ice cubes to the blender and blend again until the juice is chilled.
5. Pour the green keto energizer juice into a glass and serve immediately.

6. Enjoy your refreshing and nutritious green keto energizer juice!

Nutritional Info (per serving):

Calories: 187 | Total Fat: 15g | Saturated Fat: 2g | Cholesterol: 0mg | Sodium: 209mg | Total Carbohydrates: 14g | Dietary Fiber: 8g | Sugars: 2g | Protein: 5g

Recipe Name:________________________

Date: / / ***Time:*****____**

Rating: ☆☆☆☆☆

S/N	Ingredients	Adjustment

Cooking Experience: ______________________________

____

____

____

Notes:____________________________________

____

____

____

____

____

____

____

Berry Blast Keto Juice

Prep Time: 10 minutes
Cooking Time: 0 minutes
Servings: 1
Ingredients:

- 1/2 cup fresh strawberries
- 1/4 cup fresh blueberries
- 1/4 cup fresh raspberries
- 1/2 cup spinach leaves
- 1/2 cup unsweetened coconut water
- 1/4 cup cold water
- Ice cubes (optional)

Method of Preparation:

1. Wash the strawberries, blueberries, and raspberries.
2. In a blender, combine fresh strawberries, blueberries, raspberries, spinach leaves, unsweetened coconut water, and cold water.
3. Blend on high speed until the ingredients are well combined and the mixture is smooth.
4. If desired, add ice cubes to the blender and blend again until the juice is chilled.
5. Pour the berry blast keto juice into a glass and serve immediately.
6. Enjoy your delicious and antioxidant-rich berry blast keto juice!

Nutritional Info (per serving):
Calories: 98 | Total Fat: 1g | Saturated Fat: 0g | Cholesterol: 0mg | Sodium: 120mg | Total Carbohydrates: 24g | Dietary Fiber: 8g | Sugars: 12g | Protein: 3g

Recipe Name:________________________

Date: / / ***Time:***_____

Rating: ☆☆☆☆☆

S/N	Ingredients	Adjustment

Cooking Experience: ______________________________

Notes:____________________________________

Citrus Green Keto Juice

Prep Time: 10 minutes

Cooking Time: 0 minutes

Servings: 1

Ingredients:

- 1 cup kale leaves
- 1/2 cucumber, peeled
- 1/2 lime, peeled
- 1/2 avocado, peeled and pitted
- 1 tablespoon fresh mint leaves
- 1/2 cup unsweetened coconut water
- 1/4 cup cold water
- Ice cubes (optional)

Method of Preparation:

1. Wash the kale leaves and chop the cucumber into chunks.
2. In a blender, combine kale leaves, cucumber chunks, peeled lime, peeled avocado, fresh mint leaves, unsweetened coconut water, and cold water.
3. Blend on high speed until the ingredients are well combined and the mixture is smooth.
4. If desired, add ice cubes to the blender and blend again until the juice is chilled.
5. Pour the citrus green keto juice into a glass and serve immediately.
6. Enjoy your refreshing and vitamin-packed citrus green keto juice!

Nutritional Info (per serving):
Calories: 163 | Total Fat: 12g | Saturated Fat: 2g | Cholesterol: 0mg | Sodium: 91mg | Total Carbohydrates: 15g | Dietary Fiber: 8g | Sugars: 4g | Protein: 4g

Recipe Name:_______________________

Date: / /   ***Time:***_____

Rating: ☆☆☆☆☆

S/N	Ingredients	Adjustment

Cooking Experience: ______________________________

____

____

____

Notes:______________________________

____

____

____

____

____

____

____

Tropical Turmeric Keto Juice

Prep Time: 10 minutes

Cooking Time: 0 minutes

Servings: 1

Ingredients:

- 1/2 cup pineapple chunks
- 1/2 cup mango chunks
- 1/2 teaspoon ground turmeric
- 1/2 teaspoon grated fresh ginger
- 1/2 cup unsweetened coconut water
- 1/4 cup cold water
- Ice cubes (optional)

Method of Preparation:

1. In a blender, combine pineapple chunks, mango chunks, ground turmeric, grated fresh ginger, unsweetened coconut water, and cold water.
2. Blend on high speed until the ingredients are well combined and the mixture is smooth.
3. If desired, add ice cubes to the blender and blend again until the juice is chilled.
4. Pour the tropical turmeric keto juice into a glass and serve immediately.
5. Enjoy your exotic and anti-inflammatory tropical turmeric keto juice!

Nutritional Info (per serving):

Calories: 140 | Total Fat: 1g | Saturated Fat: 0g | Cholesterol: 0mg | Sodium: 90mg | Total Carbohydrates: 34g | Dietary Fiber: 4g | Sugars: 25g | Protein: 2g

Recipe Name:___________________________

Date: / / ***Time:***_____

Rating: ☆☆☆☆☆

S/N	Ingredients	Adjustment

Cooking Experience: ___________________________

____

____

____

Notes:___________________________

____

____

____

____

____

____

____

Refreshing Cucumber Mint Keto Juice

Prep Time: 10 minutes
Cooking Time: 0 minutes
Servings: 1
Ingredients:

- 1 large cucumber, peeled
- 1/4 cup fresh mint leaves
- 1/2 lime, peeled
- 1/2 cup spinach leaves
- 1/2 cup unsweetened coconut water
- 1/4 cup cold water
- Ice cubes (optional)

Method of Preparation:

1. Slice the peeled cucumber into chunks.
2. In a blender, combine cucumber chunks, fresh mint leaves, peeled lime, spinach leaves, unsweetened coconut water, and cold water.
3. Blend on high speed until the ingredients are well combined and the mixture is smooth.
4. If desired, add ice cubes to the blender and blend again until the juice is chilled.
5. Pour the refreshing cucumber mint keto juice into a glass and serve immediately.
6. Enjoy your hydrating and invigorating cucumber mint keto juice!

Nutritional Info (per serving):
Calories: 74 | Total Fat: 0g | Saturated Fat: 0g | Cholesterol: 0mg | Sodium: 181mg | Total Carbohydrates: 17g | Dietary Fiber: 2g | Sugars: 10g | Protein: 2g

Recipe Name:____________________________

Date: / / ***Time:***_____

Rating: ☆☆☆☆☆

S/N	Ingredients	Adjustment

Cooking Experience: ____________________________

____

____

____

Notes:____________________________

____

____

____

____

____

____

____

Berry-Licious Green Keto Juice

Prep Time: 10 minutes

Cooking Time: 0 minutes

Servings: 1

Ingredients:

- 1/2 cup kale leaves
- 1/2 cup spinach leaves
- 1/2 cup fresh strawberries
- 1/4 cup fresh blueberries
- 1/4 cup unsweetened coconut water
- 1/4 cup cold water
- Ice cubes (optional)

Method of Preparation:

1. Wash the kale leaves, spinach leaves, and berries.
2. In a blender, combine kale leaves, spinach leaves, fresh strawberries, fresh blueberries, unsweetened coconut water, and cold water.
3. Blend on high speed until the ingredients are well combined and the mixture is smooth.
4. If desired, add ice cubes to the blender and blend again until the juice is chilled.
5. Pour the berry-licious green keto juice into a glass and serve immediately.
6. Enjoy your antioxidant-rich and refreshing berry-licious green keto juice!

Nutritional Info (per serving):
Calories: 84 | Total Fat: 1g | Saturated Fat: 0g | Cholesterol: 0mg | Sodium: 35mg | Total Carbohydrates: 20g | Dietary Fiber: 5g | Sugars: 11g | Protein: 3g

Recipe Name:________________________

Date: / / ***Time:*****____**

Rating: ☆☆☆☆☆

S/N	Ingredients	Adjustment

Cooking Experience: ______________________________

____

____

____

Notes:______________________________

____

____

____

____

____

____

____

Zesty Lemon Ginger Keto Juice

Prep Time: 10 minutes
Cooking Time: 0 minutes
Servings: 1
Ingredients:

- 1/2 lemon, peeled
- 1-inch piece of fresh ginger, peeled
- 1 cup spinach leaves
- 1/2 cucumber, peeled
- 1/2 cup unsweetened coconut water
- 1/4 cup cold water
- Ice cubes (optional)

Method of Preparation:

1. Cut the peeled lemon into chunks.
2. In a blender, combine lemon chunks, fresh ginger, spinach leaves, peeled cucumber, unsweetened coconut water, and cold water.
3. Blend on high speed until the ingredients are well combined and the mixture is smooth.
4. If desired, add ice cubes to the blender and blend again until the juice is chilled.
5. Pour the zesty lemon ginger keto juice into a glass and serve immediately.
6. Enjoy your invigorating and metabolism-boosting zesty lemon ginger keto juice!

Nutritional Info (per serving):
Calories: 49 | Total Fat: 0g | Saturated Fat: 0g | Cholesterol: 0mg | Sodium: 60mg | Total Carbohydrates: 11g | Dietary Fiber: 2g | Sugars: 6g | Protein: 2g

Recipe Name:______________________________

Date: / / ***Time:***_____

Rating: ☆☆☆☆☆

S/N	Ingredients	Adjustment

Cooking Experience: ______________________________

____

____

____

Notes:______________________________

____

____

____

____

____

____

____

Creamy Coconut Green Keto Juice

Prep Time: 10 minutes

Cooking Time: 0 minutes

Servings: 1

Ingredients:

- 1/2 cup spinach leaves
- 1/2 avocado, peeled and pitted
- 1/2 cup unsweetened coconut milk
- 1/2 cup unsweetened coconut water
- 1/4 cup cold water
- Ice cubes (optional)

Method of Preparation:

1. In a blender, combine spinach leaves, peeled avocado, unsweetened coconut milk, unsweetened coconut water, and cold water.
2. Blend on high speed until the ingredients are well combined and the mixture is smooth.
3. If desired, add ice cubes to the blender and blend again until the juice is chilled.
4. Pour the creamy coconut green keto juice into a glass and serve immediately.
5. Enjoy your creamy and nourishing coconut green keto juice!

Nutritional Info (per serving):

Calories: 180 | Total Fat: 15g | Saturated Fat: 8g | Cholesterol: 0mg | Sodium: 150mg | Total Carbohydrates: 11g | Dietary Fiber: 6g | Sugars: 2g | Protein: 3g

Recipe Name:________________________

Date: / /

Time:**____**

Rating: ☆☆☆☆☆

S/N	Ingredients	Adjustment

Cooking Experience: ______________________________

____

____

____

Notes:______________________________

____

____

____

____

____

____

____

Spicy Green Keto Juice

Prep Time: 10 minutes

Cooking Time: 0 minutes

Servings: 1

Ingredients:

- 1 cup kale leaves
- 1/2 cucumber, peeled
- 1/2 green apple, cored
- 1/2 lemon, peeled
- 1-inch piece of fresh ginger, peeled
- 1/4 teaspoon cayenne pepper
- 1/2 cup cold water
- Ice cubes (optional)

Method of Preparation:

1. Wash the kale leaves and chop the cucumber into chunks.
2. Core and chop the green apple.
3. Cut the peeled lemon into chunks.
4. In a blender, combine kale leaves, cucumber chunks, green apple chunks, peeled lemon, fresh ginger, cayenne pepper, and cold water.
5. Blend on high speed until the ingredients are well combined and the mixture is smooth.
6. If desired, add ice cubes to the blender and blend again until the juice is chilled.
7. Pour the spicy green keto juice into a glass and serve immediately.
8. Enjoy your spicy and invigorating green keto juice!

Nutritional Info (per serving):
Calories: 93 | Total Fat: 1g | Saturated Fat: 0g | Cholesterol: 0mg | Sodium: 22mg | Total Carbohydrates: 22g | Dietary Fiber: 5g | Sugars: 11g | Protein: 4g

Recipe Name:______________________

Date: / /   ***Time:*****_____**

Rating: ☆☆☆☆☆

S/N	Ingredients	Adjustment

Cooking Experience: ____________________________________

____

____

____

Notes:____

____

____

____

____

____

____

____

Berry Citrus Keto Juice

Prep Time: 10 minutes
Cooking Time: 0 minutes
Servings: 1
Ingredients:

- 1/2 cup fresh strawberries
- 1/4 cup fresh raspberries
- 1/4 cup fresh blueberries
- 1/2 orange, peeled
- 1/2 lime, peeled
- 1/2 cup cold water
- Ice cubes (optional)

Method of Preparation:

1. Wash the strawberries, raspberries, and blueberries.
2. Peel the orange and lime, and cut them into chunks.
3. In a blender, combine fresh strawberries, raspberries, blueberries, orange chunks, lime chunks, and cold water.
4. Blend on high speed until the ingredients are well combined and the mixture is smooth.
5. If desired, add ice cubes to the blender and blend again until the juice is chilled.
6. Pour the berry citrus keto juice into a glass and serve immediately.
7. Enjoy your refreshing and vitamin-packed berry citrus keto juice!

Nutritional Info (per serving):
Calories: 97 | Total Fat: 1g | Saturated Fat: 0g | Cholesterol: 0mg | Sodium: 4mg | Total Carbohydrates: 24g | Dietary Fiber: 7g | Sugars: 15g | Protein: 2g

Recipe Name:____________________________

Date: / / ***Time:*****____**

Rating: ☆☆☆☆☆

S/N	Ingredients	Adjustment

Cooking Experience: ____________________________________

____

____

____

Notes:____

____

____

____

____

____

____

____

CHAPTER SEVEN

Sauces, Dressings and Condiments Recipes

Creamy Avocado Ranch Dressing

Prep Time: 10 minutes
Cooking Time: 0 minutes
Servings: 8
Ingredients:

- 1 ripe avocado, peeled and pitted
- 1/2 cup sour cream
- 1/4 cup mayonnaise
- 1 clove garlic, minced
- 2 tablespoons fresh parsley, chopped
- 2 tablespoons fresh dill, chopped
- 1 tablespoon fresh chives, chopped
- 1 tablespoon apple cider vinegar
- 1/4 cup water (adjust for desired consistency)
- Salt and pepper to taste

Method of Preparation:

1. In a blender or food processor, combine the ripe avocado, sour cream, mayonnaise, minced garlic, chopped parsley, chopped dill, chopped chives, and apple cider vinegar.
2. Blend until smooth and creamy, adding water as needed to reach your desired consistency.
3. Season with salt and pepper to taste, and blend again until well combined.

4. Transfer the creamy avocado ranch dressing to a jar or container with a lid.
5. Store in the refrigerator for up to one week.
6. Use as a delicious dressing for salads or as a dipping sauce for veggies!

Nutritional Info (per serving - 2 tablespoons):
Calories: 101 | Total Fat: 10g | Saturated Fat: 3g | Cholesterol: 10mg | Sodium: 68mg | Total Carbohydrates: 2g | Dietary Fiber: 1g | Sugars: 0g | Protein: 1g

Recipe Name:_______________________

Date: / /   ***Time:*____**

Rating: ☆☆☆☆☆

S/N	Ingredients	Adjustment

Cooking Experience: ______________________________

____

____

____

Notes:____________________________________

____

____

____

____

____

____

____

Garlic Parmesan Zucchini Noodles

Prep Time: 10 minutes

Cooking Time: 10 minutes

Servings: 4

Ingredients:

- 4 medium zucchinis
- 2 tablespoons olive oil
- 2 cloves garlic, minced
- 1/4 cup grated Parmesan cheese
- Salt and pepper to taste
- Fresh parsley, chopped for garnish

Method of Preparation:

1. Trim the ends of the zucchinis and spiralize them into noodles using a spiralizer.
2. Heat olive oil in a large skillet over medium heat. Add the minced garlic and cook until fragrant, about 1 minute.
3. Add the zucchini noodles to the skillet and toss to coat them in the garlic-infused oil. Cook for 3-4 minutes, stirring occasionally, until the noodles are tender but still slightly crisp.
4. Remove the skillet from the heat and sprinkle the grated Parmesan cheese over the zucchini noodles. Toss to combine until the cheese is melted and coats the noodles evenly.
5. Season with salt and pepper to taste.
6. Transfer the garlic Parmesan zucchini noodles to a serving dish and garnish with chopped fresh parsley.
7. Serve immediately as a flavorful low-carb alternative to pasta!

Nutritional Info (per serving):
Calories: 94 | Total Fat: 7g | Saturated Fat: 2g | Cholesterol: 5mg | Sodium: 102mg | Total Carbohydrates: 6g | Dietary Fiber: 2g | Sugars: 3g | Protein: 3g

Recipe Name:________________________

Date: / / ***Time:***_____

Rating: ☆☆☆☆☆

S/N	Ingredients	Adjustment

Cooking Experience: ______________________________

____

____

____

Notes:____________________________________

____

____

____

____

____

____

____

Keto Pesto Sauce

Prep Time: 10 minutes

Cooking Time: 0 minutes

Servings: 8

Ingredients:

- 2 cups fresh basil leaves, packed
- 1/2 cup grated Parmesan cheese
- 1/4 cup pine nuts
- 2 cloves garlic
- 1/2 cup extra virgin olive oil
- Salt and pepper to taste

Method of Preparation:

1. In a food processor, combine the fresh basil leaves, grated Parmesan cheese, pine nuts, and garlic cloves.
2. Pulse until the ingredients are finely chopped and well combined.
3. While the food processor is running, slowly drizzle in the extra virgin olive oil until the mixture forms a smooth paste.
4. Season with salt and pepper to taste, and pulse a few more times to incorporate.
5. Transfer the keto pesto sauce to a jar or container with a lid.
6. Store in the refrigerator for up to one week.
7. Use as a delicious sauce for zucchini noodles, grilled chicken, or as a topping for low-carb pizzas!

Nutritional Info (per serving - 2 tablespoons):
Calories: 163 | Total Fat: 17g | Saturated Fat: 3g | Cholesterol: 4mg | Sodium: 93mg | Total Carbohydrates: 1g | Dietary Fiber: 0g | Sugars: 0g | Protein: 2g

Recipe Name:____________________

Date: / /　　　　***Time:***_____

Rating: ☆☆☆☆☆

S/N	Ingredients	Adjustment

Cooking Experience: ____________________

____

____

____

Notes:____________________

____

____

____

____

____

____

____

Low-Carb Buffalo Wing Sauce

Prep Time: 5 minutes

Cooking Time: 10 minutes

Servings: 8

Ingredients:

- 1/2 cup unsalted butter
- 1/2 cup hot sauce (such as Frank's RedHot)
- 1 tablespoon Worcestershire sauce
- 1 teaspoon garlic powder
- 1/2 teaspoon onion powder
- Salt to taste

Method of Preparation:

1. In a small saucepan, melt the unsalted butter over medium-low heat.
2. Once the butter is melted, add the hot sauce, Worcestershire sauce, garlic powder, and onion powder to the saucepan.
3. Stir the mixture until all the ingredients are well combined.
4. Bring the sauce to a simmer and let it cook for 5-10 minutes, stirring occasionally, until it thickens slightly.
5. Remove the saucepan from the heat and let the buffalo wing sauce cool for a few minutes.
6. Taste and adjust seasoning with salt if needed.
7. Transfer the low-carb buffalo wing sauce to a jar or container with a lid.
8. Use immediately as a dipping sauce for chicken wings or drizzle it over grilled meats for a spicy kick!

Nutritional Info (per serving - 2 tablespoons):
Calories: 102 | Total Fat: 11g | Saturated Fat: 7g | Cholesterol: 31mg | Sodium: 751mg | Total Carbohydrates: 1g | Dietary Fiber: 0g | Sugars: 0g | Protein: 0g

Recipe Name:________________________

Date: / /

Time:_____

Rating: ☆☆☆☆☆

S/N	Ingredients	Adjustment

Cooking Experience: ________________________________

____

____

____

Notes:________________________________

____

____

____

____

____

____

____

Keto Caesar Dressing

Prep Time: 10 minutes

Cooking Time: 0 minutes

Servings: 8

Ingredients:

- 1/2 cup mayonnaise
- 2 tablespoons grated Parmesan cheese
- 2 tablespoons lemon juice
- 1 tablespoon Dijon mustard
- 1 clove garlic, minced
- 1/2 teaspoon Worcestershire sauce
- Salt and pepper to taste

Method of Preparation:

1. In a mixing bowl, combine mayonnaise, grated Parmesan cheese, lemon juice, Dijon mustard, minced garlic, and Worcestershire sauce.
2. Whisk until all the ingredients are well combined and the mixture is smooth.
3. Season with salt and pepper to taste, and whisk again to incorporate.
4. Transfer the keto Caesar dressing to a jar or container with a lid.
5. Store in the refrigerator for up to one week.
6. Use as a classic dressing for Caesar salads or as a dip for fresh veggies!

Nutritional Info (per serving - 2 tablespoons):
Calories: 121 | Total Fat: 13g | Saturated Fat: 2g | Cholesterol: 7mg | Sodium: 169mg | Total Carbohydrates: 1g | Dietary Fiber: 0g | Sugars: 0g | Protein: 1g

Recipe Name:______________________

Date: / /   ***Time:***_____

Rating: ☆☆☆☆☆

S/N	Ingredients	Adjustment

Cooking Experience: ______________________________

____

____

____

Notes:______________________________

____

____

____

____

____

____

____

Keto Tomato Basil Sauce

Prep Time: 10 minutes

Cooking Time: 20 minutes

Servings: 8

Ingredients:

- 2 tablespoons olive oil
- 2 cloves garlic, minced
- 1/4 teaspoon red pepper flakes (optional)
- 1 (28-ounce) can crushed tomatoes
- 2 tablespoons tomato paste
- 1 teaspoon dried basil
- 1/2 teaspoon dried oregano
- Salt and pepper to taste
- Fresh basil leaves, chopped for garnish (optional)

Method of Preparation:

1. Heat olive oil in a saucepan over medium heat. Add minced garlic and red pepper flakes (if using), and sauté for 1-2 minutes until fragrant.
2. Stir in crushed tomatoes, tomato paste, dried basil, and dried oregano.
3. Season with salt and pepper to taste, and stir until well combined.
4. Bring the sauce to a simmer, then reduce the heat to low and let it simmer gently for 15-20 minutes, stirring occasionally, until the sauce thickens.
5. Remove the saucepan from the heat and let the keto tomato basil sauce cool for a few minutes.
6. Taste and adjust seasoning if needed.
7. Garnish with chopped fresh basil leaves if desired.

8. Serve the keto tomato basil sauce over zucchini noodles or grilled chicken for a delicious low-carb meal!

Nutritional Info (per serving - 1/2 cup):
Calories: 52 | Total Fat: 3g | Saturated Fat: 0g | Cholesterol: 0mg | Sodium: 150mg | Total Carbohydrates: 6g | Dietary Fiber: 2g | Sugars: 4g | Protein: 2g

Recipe Name:___________________________

Date: / / ***Time:***_____

Rating: ☆☆☆☆☆

S/N	Ingredients	Adjustment

Cooking Experience: ______________________________

____

____

____

Notes:______________________________

____

____

____

____

____

____

____

Keto Blue Cheese Dressing

Prep Time: 10 minutes

Cooking Time: 0 minutes

Servings: 8

Ingredients:

- 1/2 cup mayonnaise
- 1/4 cup sour cream
- 2 ounces blue cheese, crumbled
- 1 tablespoon lemon juice
- 1 clove garlic, minced
- 1/4 teaspoon Worcestershire sauce
- Salt and pepper to taste

Method of Preparation:

1. In a mixing bowl, combine mayonnaise, sour cream, crumbled blue cheese, lemon juice, minced garlic, and Worcestershire sauce.
2. Mix until all the ingredients are well combined and the mixture is smooth.
3. Season with salt and pepper to taste, and mix again to incorporate.
4. Transfer the keto blue cheese dressing to a jar or container with a lid.
5. Store in the refrigerator for up to one week.
6. Use as a flavorful dressing for salads or as a dip for buffalo cauliflower bites!

Nutritional Info (per serving - 2 tablespoons):
Calories: 138 | Total Fat: 14g | Saturated Fat: 4g | Cholesterol: 17mg | Sodium: 191mg | Total Carbohydrates: 1g | Dietary Fiber: 0g | Sugars: 0g | Protein: 2g

Recipe Name:______________________________

Date: / / ***Time:***_____

Rating: ☆☆☆☆☆

S/N	Ingredients	Adjustment

Cooking Experience: ______________________________

____

____

____

Notes:______________________________

____

____

____

____

____

____

____

Keto Balsamic Vinaigrette

Prep Time: 5 minutes

Cooking Time: 0 minutes

Servings: 8

Ingredients:

- 1/4 cup balsamic vinegar
- 1/4 cup extra virgin olive oil
- 1 tablespoon Dijon mustard
- 1 clove garlic, minced
- 1/2 teaspoon dried oregano
- Salt and pepper to taste

Method of Preparation:

1. In a small bowl, whisk together balsamic vinegar, extra virgin olive oil, Dijon mustard, minced garlic, and dried oregano.
2. Continue whisking until the ingredients are emulsified and the vinaigrette is well combined.
3. Season with salt and pepper to taste, and whisk again to incorporate.
4. Transfer the keto balsamic vinaigrette to a jar or container with a lid.
5. Store in the refrigerator for up to one week.
6. Use as a tangy dressing for salads or as a marinade for grilled vegetables!

Nutritional Info (per serving - 2 tablespoons):
Calories: 107 | Total Fat: 11g | Saturated Fat: 1g | Cholesterol: 0mg | Sodium: 60mg | Total Carbohydrates: 1g | Dietary Fiber: 0g | Sugars: 1g | Protein: 0g

Recipe Name:______________________

Date: / /   ***Time:***____

Rating: ☆☆☆☆☆

S/N	Ingredients	Adjustment

Cooking Experience: ______________________________

____

____

____

Notes:______________________________

____

____

____

____

____

____

____

Keto Creamy Garlic Sauce

Prep Time: 5 minutes

Cooking Time: 10 minutes

Servings: 8

Ingredients:

- 2 tablespoons unsalted butter
- 4 cloves garlic, minced
- 1 cup heavy cream
- 1/4 cup grated Parmesan cheese
- 1 teaspoon Italian seasoning
- Salt and pepper to taste
- Chopped fresh parsley for garnish (optional)

Method of Preparation:

1. In a saucepan, melt the unsalted butter over medium heat.
2. Add the minced garlic to the saucepan and sauté for 1-2 minutes until fragrant.
3. Pour in the heavy cream and bring it to a simmer, stirring occasionally.
4. Reduce the heat to low and simmer the cream for 5-7 minutes until it thickens slightly.
5. Stir in the grated Parmesan cheese and Italian seasoning until the cheese is melted and the sauce is smooth.
6. Season with salt and pepper to taste.
7. Remove the saucepan from the heat and let the keto creamy garlic sauce cool for a few minutes.
8. Garnish with chopped fresh parsley if desired.
9. Serve the creamy garlic sauce over grilled chicken, steamed vegetables, or zucchini noodles for a decadent low-carb meal!

Nutritional Info (per serving - 2 tablespoons):
Calories: 144 | Total Fat: 15g | Saturated Fat: 9g | Cholesterol: 51mg | Sodium: 51mg | Total Carbohydrates: 1g | Dietary Fiber: 0g | Sugars: 0g | Protein: 1g

Recipe Name:________________________

Date: / / ***Time:***_____

Rating: ☆☆☆☆☆

S/N	Ingredients	Adjustment

Cooking Experience: ______________________________

____

____

____

Notes:_____________________________________

____

____

____

____

____

____

____

Keto Chipotle Mayo

Prep Time: 5 minutes

Cooking Time: 0 minutes

Servings: 8

Ingredients:

- 1/2 cup mayonnaise
- 2 tablespoons chipotle peppers in adobo sauce, minced
- 1 tablespoon lime juice
- 1 teaspoon smoked paprika
- Salt to taste

Method of Preparation:

1. In a small bowl, combine mayonnaise, minced chipotle peppers in adobo sauce, lime juice, and smoked paprika.
2. Stir until all the ingredients are well combined.
3. Season with salt to taste, and stir again to incorporate.
4. Transfer the keto chipotle mayo to a jar or container with a lid.
5. Store in the refrigerator for up to one week.
6. Use as a spicy spread for sandwiches, burgers, or as a dip for sweet potato fries!

Nutritional Info (per serving - 2 tablespoons):
Calories: 106 | Total Fat: 11g | Saturated Fat: 2g | Cholesterol: 8mg | Sodium: 178mg | Total Carbohydrates: 1g | Dietary Fiber: 0g | Sugars: 0g | Protein: 0g

Recipe Name:______________________________

Date: / / ***Time:*****_____**

Rating: ☆☆☆☆☆

S/N	Ingredients	Adjustment

Cooking Experience: ______________________________

____

____

____

Notes:______________________________

____

____

____

____

____

____

____

CHAPTER EIGHT

Navigating Challenges on the Keto Journey

Starting a keto diet may be an exciting path to better health, more energy, and weight loss. However, like with any dietary shift, it has its own set of obstacles. From managing cravings to comprehending keto flu symptoms, newbies frequently encounter roadblocks that make adhering to the diet challenging. But do not worry, since with the correct information and tactics, you can overcome these obstacles and flourish on the keto diet. In this chapter, we'll look at some of the most frequent challenges that people have while starting the keto diet, as well as practical answers and recommendations to help you succeed.

Understanding Keto Flu

The dreaded keto flu is one of the most common obstacles that newbies to the keto diet confront. This transitory set of symptoms might appear within the first few days or weeks of beginning the diet as your body adjusts to using fat for fuel rather than carbs. Keto flu symptoms may include tiredness, headache, dizziness, nausea, irritability, and problems focusing.

Solution: To alleviate the symptoms of keto flu, remain hydrated and restore electrolytes. Drink lots of water throughout the day, and include electrolyte-rich foods like leafy greens, avocados, nuts, and seeds in your meals. You can also supplement with electrolyte drinks or powders to assist keep your electrolytes balanced. Be patient with your body while it adjusts to the new dietary adjustments, and remember that keto flu symptoms usually resolve within a week or two.

Dealing with Cravings

Many beginners on the keto diet struggle with cravings for high-carb items. Cravings, whether they're for sweet goodies or starchy snacks, may derail even the most well-intentioned keto dieter.

Solution: To combat cravings, focus on rewarding keto-friendly alternatives. To satisfy hunger between meals, keep low-carb snacks on hand, such as almonds, cheese, olives, and pork rinds. Incorporate fragrant herbs and spices into your cooking to improve the flavor of keto-friendly recipes. Consider adopting mindful eating strategies to become more aware of your body's hunger and satiety signals. Remember that cravings are just transitory and will fade over time as your body adjusts to the keto diet.

Navigating Social Situations

Eating out or attending social events may be difficult for keto newbies, especially when there is a limited variety of keto-friendly alternatives or peer pressure to eat high-carb foods.

Solution: Before going out to eat or attending social gatherings, have a plan and conduct research. Look for keto-friendly menu selections online, or call ahead to ask about replacements or changes. If you're going to a picnic or event, bring a keto-friendly meal to share with everyone. Don't be afraid to gently refuse things that don't fit your nutritional objectives, and instead enjoy the company of friends and family.

Overcoming Plateaus

It's not unusual for keto newbies to hit weight reduction plateaus, in which the scale appears to stall despite following the diet.

Solution: If you reach a plateau, don't be disheartened. Plateaus are a normal part of the weight reduction process and can usually be overcome with patience and perseverance. Consider reassessing your eating habits and measuring your food consumption to ensure you're remaining within your macronutrient limits. To kickstart your metabolism, try intermittent fasting or a new workout plan. Remember that weight reduction is not always linear, so focus on non-scale successes like more energy, improved attitude, and better-fitting apparel.

Seeking Support and Accountability

Starting the keto journey may be stressful, especially when met with hurdles along the road. Having a support system in place may make a significant difference in keeping motivated and responsible to your goals.

Solution: Seek support from friends, family, or online communities that are also on the keto diet. Share your accomplishments, challenges, and questions with others who can provide support and guidance. To keep on track, consider working with an accountability partner or joining a keto-focused club or forum. Remember that you are not alone in this path, and having a supporting network may be a source of important encouragement and drive.

To summarize, while beginning the keto diet might be difficult, with the appropriate tactics and mentality, you can overcome these problems and thrive on your keto adventure. Understanding keto flu symptoms, controlling cravings, preparing ahead for social settings, overcoming weight loss plateaus, and seeking support from others can set you up for success on your journey to a healthy, low-carb lifestyle. Stay focused, dedicated, and enjoy the path to a happier, healthier self.

30-DAY MEAL PLAN

Day	Breakfast	Lunch	Dinner	Snack
1	Zesty Lemon Ginger Keto Juice	Creamy Avocado Ranch Dressing with Salad	Garlic Parmesan Zucchini Noodles	Keto Blue Cheese Dressing with Veggies
2	Creamy Coconut Green Keto Juice	Spicy Green Keto Juice	Low-Carb Buffalo Wing Sauce with Chicken	Keto Pesto Sauce with Veggies
3	Berry Citrus Keto Juice	Keto Caesar Salad with Grilled Chicken	Keto Chipotle Mayo with Lettuce Wraps	Almonds
4	Zesty Lemon Ginger Keto Juice	Creamy Avocado Ranch Dressing with Salad	Garlic Parmesan Zucchini Noodles	Keto Blue Cheese Dressing with Veggies
5	Creamy Coconut Green Keto Juice	Spicy Green Keto Juice	Low-Carb Buffalo Wing Sauce with Chicken	Keto Pesto Sauce with Veggies
6	Berry Citrus Keto Juice	Keto Caesar Salad with Grilled Chicken	Keto Chipotle Mayo with Lettuce Wraps	Almonds
7	Zesty Lemon Ginger Keto Juice	Creamy Avocado Ranch Dressing with Salad	Garlic Parmesan Zucchini Noodles	Keto Blue Cheese Dressing with Veggies

8	Creamy Coconut Green Keto Juice	Spicy Green Keto Juice	Low-Carb Buffalo Wing Sauce with Chicken	Keto Pesto Sauce with Veggies
9	Berry Citrus Keto Juice	Keto Caesar Salad with Grilled Chicken	Keto Chipotle Mayo with Lettuce Wraps	Almonds
10	Zesty Lemon Ginger Keto Juice	Creamy Avocado Ranch Dressing with Salad	Garlic Parmesan Zucchini Noodles	Keto Blue Cheese Dressing with Veggies
11	Creamy Coconut Green Keto Juice	Spicy Green Keto Juice	Low-Carb Buffalo Wing Sauce with Chicken	Keto Pesto Sauce with Veggies
12	Berry Citrus Keto Juice	Keto Caesar Salad with Grilled Chicken	Keto Chipotle Mayo with Lettuce Wraps	Almonds
13	Zesty Lemon Ginger Keto Juice	Creamy Avocado Ranch Dressing with Salad	Garlic Parmesan Zucchini Noodles	Keto Blue Cheese Dressing with Veggies
14	Creamy Coconut Green Keto Juice	Spicy Green Keto Juice	Low-Carb Buffalo Wing Sauce with Chicken	Keto Pesto Sauce with Veggies
15	Berry Citrus Keto Juice	Keto Caesar Salad with Grilled Chicken	Keto Chipotle Mayo with Lettuce Wraps	Almonds

16	Zesty Lemon Ginger Keto Juice	Creamy Avocado Ranch Dressing with Salad	Garlic Parmesan Zucchini Noodles	Keto Blue Cheese Dressing with Veggies
17	Creamy Coconut Green Keto Juice	Spicy Green Keto Juice	Low-Carb Buffalo Wing Sauce with Chicken	Keto Pesto Sauce with Veggies
18	Berry Citrus Keto Juice	Keto Caesar Salad with Grilled Chicken	Keto Chipotle Mayo with Lettuce Wraps	Almonds
19	Zesty Lemon Ginger Keto Juice	Creamy Avocado Ranch Dressing with Salad	Garlic Parmesan Zucchini Noodles	Keto Blue Cheese Dressing with Veggies
20	Creamy Coconut Green Keto Juice	Spicy Green Keto Juice	Low-Carb Buffalo Wing Sauce with Chicken	Keto Pesto Sauce with Veggies
21	Berry Citrus Keto Juice	Keto Caesar Salad with Grilled Chicken	Keto Chipotle Mayo with Lettuce Wraps	Almonds
22	Zesty Lemon Ginger Keto Juice	Creamy Avocado Ranch Dressing with Salad	Garlic Parmesan Zucchini Noodles	Keto Blue Cheese Dressing with Veggies
23	Creamy Coconut Green Keto Juice	Spicy Green Keto Juice	Low-Carb Buffalo Wing Sauce with Chicken	Keto Pesto Sauce with Veggies

24	Berry Citrus Keto Juice	Keto Caesar Salad with Grilled Chicken	Keto Chipotle Mayo with Lettuce Wraps	Almonds
25	Zesty Lemon Ginger Keto Juice	Creamy Avocado Ranch Dressing with Salad	Garlic Parmesan Zucchini Noodles	Keto Blue Cheese Dressing with Veggies
26	Creamy Coconut Green Keto Juice	Spicy Green Keto Juice	Low-Carb Buffalo Wing Sauce with Chicken	Keto Pesto Sauce with Veggies
27	Berry Citrus Keto Juice	Keto Caesar Salad with Grilled Chicken	Keto Chipotle Mayo with Lettuce Wraps	Almonds
28	Zesty Lemon Ginger Keto Juice	Creamy Avocado Ranch Dressing with Salad	Garlic Parmesan Zucchini Noodles	Keto Blue Cheese Dressing with Veggies
29	Creamy Coconut Green Keto Juice	Spicy Green Keto Juice	Low-Carb Buffalo Wing Sauce with Chicken	Keto Pesto Sauce with Veggies
30	Berry Citrus Keto Juice	Keto Caesar Salad with Grilled Chicken	Keto Chipotle Mayo with Lettuce Wraps	Almonds

This meal plan provides a variety of delicious and nutritious keto-friendly options to keep you satisfied and on track with your dietary goals. Remember to adjust portion sizes and ingredients based on your individual caloric and macronutrient needs. Enjoy your journey to better health with these flavorful keto recipes!

CONCLUSION

In this comprehensive guide, "The Complete Keto Diet Cookbook for Beginners 2024," we've set out on a road to a healthier, lower-carb living. We've explored the world of ketogenic eating with a wealth of tasty recipes, smart explanations, and practical suggestions, and we've given ourselves the skills we need to flourish on this transforming diet.

Throughout this book, we've debunked the keto diet by delving into its core ideas and metabolic pathways. We've built the framework for keto success by understanding the metabolic mechanism of ketosis as well as the importance of macronutrients such as fat, protein, and carbohydrates. We've learned how to measure and track our nutritional intake, allowing us to make informed decisions that support our health and wellness goals.

Beyond mere theory, this cookbook has brought the keto diet to life with a delectable collection of meals. From vivid breakfast drinks to meaty supper dinners and filling snacks, each item has been thoughtfully designed to delight the taste senses while complementing our low-carb lifestyle. Whether it's creamy avocado ranch dressing, garlic parmesan zucchini noodles, or keto-friendly sweets, we've realized that eating keto doesn't have to mean giving up flavor or enjoyment.

However, the keto path is not without its hurdles. From navigating keto flu symptoms to managing cravings and breaking through weight loss plateaus, we faced challenges head on and emerged stronger and more resilient. We've learned to handle the ups and downs of the keto diet with grace and resolve by implementing practical tactics like staying hydrated, getting support from our keto network, and practicing mindful eating.

As we wrap off our investigation of the keto diet, consider its transforming power. The keto diet has other benefits in addition to weight reduction, including increased energy and mental clarity, as well as better metabolic health and longevity. By adopting the keto diet, we are not only altering what we consume, but also reshaping our lives from inside.

So, to everyone starting out on their ketogenic path, I give these words of support and motivation. Accept the adventure with an open heart and an inquisitive mind. Celebrate minor accomplishments along the road, such as fitting into your favorite pair of pants or mastering a new keto dish. Remember that growth is not always linear, and setbacks are a normal part of the process. But with endurance, commitment, and a dash of imagination, you can reach your health and fitness objectives.

Above all, embrace the keto diet with positivity and thankfulness. Enjoy the great tastes, wholesome ingredients, and renewed energy that each keto meal provides. Most importantly, embrace the trip itself—the moments of self-discovery, triumph over hardship, and relationships formed with other keto aficionados along the road.

As you begin on this changing journey, may each mouthful bring you joy, contentment, and plenty. Wishing you health, happiness, and success on your ketogenic journey. Bon appétit, and keto on!

Printed in Great Britain
by Amazon